DRUG
MONITORING
AND
PHARMACOKINETIC DATA

Hugo C. Pribor, M.D., Ph.D.
George Morrell, M.S.
George H. Scherr, Ph.D.

1980

PATHOTOX PUBLISHERS, INC.
2405 Bond Street, Park Forest South, Illinois 60466
U.S.A.

PATHOTOX PUBLISHERS, INC.
2405 Bond Street, Park Forest South, Illinois 60466

Library of Congress Catalog Card Number:79-90657
ISBN 0-930376-10-2

Printed in The United States of America

TO ALL THOSE WHO LABOR TO
PRESERVE LIFE AND DIGNITY AND
ARE UNHERALDED BECAUSE THEY
SERVE HUMBLY.

DRUG MONITORING
AND
PHARMACOKINETIC DATA

TABLE OF CONTENTS

TABLES

TABLES

FIGURES

ACKNOWLEDGEMENTS

We appreciate the courtesies of:

Dynatech Laboratories, Inc., for the use of the photograph of their MIC-2000 instrument (Figure 7).

Difco Laboratories for the use of the photograph of their Disc Dispenser (Figure 6).

Science Spectrum for the use of the photograph of their Differential III instrument (Figure 8).

Pfizer Diagnostics Division for the use of the photograph of their "Autobac" instrument (Figure 9).

Data used in Tables and other Figures are acknowleged in the text where pertinent.

Is there then any such happiness as for a man's mind to be raised above the confusion of things, where he may have a respect of the order of nature and the error of men? Is there but a view only of delight and not of discovery? Of contentment and not of benefit? Shall we not discern as well the riches of nature's warehouse as the beauty of her shop? Is truth barren? Shall we not thereby be able to produce worthy effects, and to endow the life of man with infinite commodities?

from the Praise of Knowledge
by Francis Bacon

Preface

The purpose of this book is to provide clinicians and laboratorians with a ready reference guide to establish therapeutic as well as toxic levels of drugs which may be readily monitored in the laboratory with concomitant citations of the clinical signs of drug toxicity. We have conceived this guide as a single source of informative material for the clinician and/or other laboratory professionals involved in the rapidly expanding field of therapeutic drug monitoring. While the cookbook approach to therapeutic drug monitoring, particularly when citing therapeutic dose ranges and toxicity symptomology, may be somewhat misleading, we feel that presenting these data in a single source combined with interpretive information and actual case histories, can provide the necessary supportive information to complement the factual listings of the various tables and charts. In practice, therefore, a clinician or pathologist may readily determine the generic and/or brand names of a compound, various pharmacokinetic and pharmacologic properties of that particular compound, along with dosage information and approximate therapeutic serum or plasma levels. However, a caveat is in order—all personnel utilizing the information contained herein must realize that therapeutic drug monitoring only exists and only provides an equitable method for the clinician to evaluate patient response to therapy with the combined use of a detailed clinical history. One must always realize that there are exceptions to all the rules, ranges and other data presented and that each patient responds quite differently to a given standard dose of any medication due to genetic, physiological, psychological, and pathological factors.

A particularly frustrating problem for the clinician is the prescribing of selected "adequate" therapy, only to observe a lack of therapeutic response. A few years ago the measurement of plasma levels of various drugs was principally a research tool; currently, the monitoring of serum or plasma levels of chemotherapeutic agents has become part of routine management of patients. The rapid expansion of the practice of managing various disease states in relation to serum or drug plasma levels has occurred before there has been sufficient time for a thorough exploration of their correlation with clinical results and pharmacokinetic considerations. This book is therefore intended to assess and bring together in a single monograph the various data available for chemotherapeutic drug monitoring.

While prevailing thought in the scientific community has evolved more towards the use of a standardized generic listing for various drugs, we find in practice, particularly in the hospital environment, that the use of brand names is still in widespread use. For continuity throughout this text, we have relegated to the use of generic terminology. However, as a ready guide to professional personnel in order to provide a more useful utilization of this text in those environments where brand names are still being extensively utilized, we have listed an extensive table cross-referencing the various brand and registered trade names to the appropriate generic terminology.

To the best of our knowledge, the data contained herein is accurate and was arrived at by a review of many compendia and reports, as well as personal data. We would appreciate being advised of any misinformation, errors, or update of data that the readers feel have been omitted or overlooked in the text so that we can in future editions update the information provided in this text to assure the professional community of current state-of-the-art citations of the various pharmacokinetic and pharmacologic data outlined herein.

Standard dosages and other pharmacokinetic and pharmacologic data here presented have been adapted from various standardized texts as noted in the cited references. However, these data are to be used only as guidelines to allow the clinician and the practicing professional to compile the various data necessary for a more complete understanding of their ramifications for therapeutic drug monitoring. These are not intended to be a rigorous approach to administration of medication nor are they intended to imply that they may be the same for all patients. The package insert for each drug should be consulted for use of dosages as approved by the U.S. Food and Drug Administration or other regulatory agencies. We feel an excellent source of dosage data to be the annual publication of the PDR and its supplementary information produced throughout the year. As noted by Bochner and associates (1978), "prescribing a drug involves little mental or physical effort—to do it badly! A little more effort may produce considerable benefits for the individual patients and for society."

Hugo C. Pribor, M.D., Ph.D.
George Morrell, M.S.
George H. Scherr, Ph.D.

1. Introduction

The enormous differences in pharmacologic action found in individuals following a single dose of a drug are not surprising when one considers the innumerable factors that effect a drug's actions (Figure 1). It is not generally appreciated that the variability of the dose-effect relation among different patients is primarily due to individual differences in the serum and/or tissue concentrations achieved with a given dosage schedule rather than to different modes of action that could be attributable to the same serum concentrations (Pippenger et al., 1978; Morrell and Pribor, 1977).

The relation between dosage of a drug and its concentration in the serum will be influenced by the bioavailability of the dosage form used, by host factors that affect the degree of gastrointestinal absorption, by body size and composition, by distribution through fluid compartments, by binding at various sites, and by rates of metabolism and excretion. All these determinants are subject to much individual variation due to genetic and environmental factors, to consequences of disease, and to concomitant administration of other drugs (Brodie, 1967). Individual variation in the rate of drug elimination is quantitatively most important. There are significant genetically controlled differences due to induction or inhibition of drug-metabolizing enzyme systems. For example, a quantative variation from person to person of the activity of human serum cholinesterase has been frequently observed. There also exists a qualitative variation of the enzyme activity which finds its expression in differences of substrate specificity and susceptibility to inhibition. Genetic studies undertaken thus far have shown the gene for a typical cholinesterase to have widespread distribution throughout the world.

Cholinesterase catabolizes several drugs used in anesthesia and is responsible for the very brief effect of muscle relaxant succinylcholine, due to the drug's rapid metabolic degradation by cholinesterase. The degradative reaction is a simple hydrolysis to the pharmacologically inert succinylmonocholine. A patient with abnormal cholinesterase or very little cholinesterase is not able to metabolize this drug effectively, and occasionally such patients manifest a bizarre response to succinylcholine: prolonged muscular relaxation and apnea lasting as long as several hours after discontinuance of the infusion (Kalow, 1956).

Farfel and his coworkers (1978a, 1978b) have reported a syndrome of hyperkalaemia hypertension in 7 members of a given family ranging in age from 4 to 56, over an expanse of three generations. The pattern of inheritance suggested autosomal dominance, and was again characterized by excellent response to a benzothiadiazine (chorothiazide). These workers suggested that the disorder was not simply an isolated renal tubular transport deficiency, but a generalized cell membrane defect that specifically impedes potassium influx. Lee and Morgan (1980) reported the existence of this syndrome and supported the view that even slight over-reabsorption of sodium (together with potassium) may lead to a syndrome indistinguishable from essential hypertension with a

4

FIGURE 1[1]

DOSE-EFFECT RELATION OF DRUGS IN MAN AND THE FACTORS THAT INFLUENCE IT.

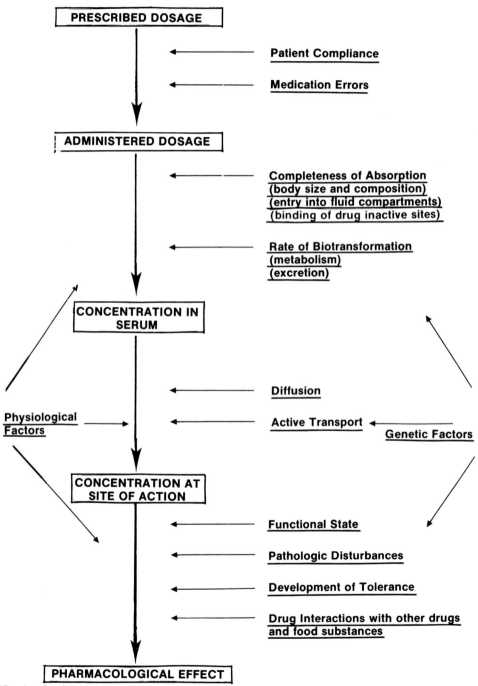

PRESCRIBED DOSAGE

Patient Compliance

Medication Errors

ADMINISTERED DOSAGE

Completeness of Absorption
(body size and composition)
(entry into fluid compartments)
(binding of drug inactive sites)

Rate of Biotransformation
(metabolism)
(excretion)

CONCENTRATION IN SERUM

Diffusion

Physiological Factors

Active Transport

Genetic Factors

CONCENTRATION AT SITE OF ACTION

Functional State

Pathologic Disturbances

Development of Tolerance

Drug Interactions with other drugs and food substances

PHARMACOLOGICAL EFFECT

[1]Reprinted with permission from Laboratory Management, Morrell and Pribor, Vol 16, No 7, July, 1978, pg 15-27.

low plasma renin activity (PRA). They concluded "hypertensive patients with low PRA's have a higher total of extinguishable body sodium and a somewhat higher total exchangeable potassium then hypertensives with normal PRA. Perhaps these two patients represent an extreme example of a renal tubular (or membrane) disorder which could result, in a less extreme form, in asymtomatic essential hypertension. This could also explain why some patients with essential hypertension show a marked fall of arterial pressure when given benzothiadiazine diuretics." It appears, therefore, that there is a familial (genetic) response to benzothiadizine diuretic administration—another poignant example of genetic preinformation clarifying the response to various drugs. (Woods et al., 1969).

Additional hereditary characters whose presence have been shown to enhance the risk to various drug reactions include erythrocyte deficiency in methhemoglobin which may cause increased risk of drug reactions following the administration of sulfonamides or various nitrates and amines (Cawein et al., 1964; Kalow, 1962). The hemoglobin H variant may also increase the risk of toxicity following administration of sulfonamides or nitrites (Rigas and Koler, 1961). The Crigler-Najjer syndrome, a deficiency in hepatic glucuronyl transferase, may result in possible potentiation of toxicity following adminstration salicylates. Also, hepatic porphyria, has been shown to increase the potentiation of drug reactions (Tschudy, 1968) with the administration of barbiturates due to an increased porphyrin synthesis.

Disease-induced disturbances in cardiac, hepatic, and renal function are also responsible for much variation in the biologic half-life of drugs (Brodie and Reid, 1971). Dettli(Dettli et al., 1971; Dettli, 1974) has postulated that the following therapeutic approach should be taken for a patient with impaired renal function: "The drug level resulting in the patient with renal disease should be the same and should be reached after a similar time interval as in patients with normal renal function." He has enumerated two steps that may be reached without measuring the drug plasma concentrations if the following have been addressed:

1. A quantitative relationship between a simple routine test of function on the one hand and the speed of drug elimination on the the other must be determined experimentally in the representative sample of patients with renal disease.
2. Based on the estimated elimination rate, a modified dosage regime of the drug for each individual patient must be calculated according to various pharmacokinetic principles.

It was stressed that uremic patients should be carefully watched for signs of unexpected drug toxicity and when a relatively toxic drug which is eliminated almost entirely by the kidneys is administered to a patient with severe renal impairment, even small deviations from the estimated elimination rate caused by biological variability may result in toxic drug accumulation (Reidenberg, 1971). Under these circumstances the safe and effective use of the drug may depend on the measurement of serum concentration, particularly in the case of aminoglycosides, for example, gentamicin and tobramycin.

Individual differences also exist in the processes that determine the relation between the serum drug level, concentration at the site of drug action, and efficacy of drug action. Thus, *serum concentrations of drugs are not perfect indices of the degree of pharmacologic response.* The important point is that a more accurate prediction of pharmacologic response can be made for many drugs from the serum level than from the prescribed dosage. By determining serum concentrations, one at least eliminates the largest source of individual differences in the dose-pharmacologic relationship of therapeutic drugs. For this reason, dosage adjustments can often be guided by knowledge of serum levels (Vessell and Passananti, 1971).

Measurements of serum levels of drugs become useful guides for dosage adjustments only when the therapeutically effective range of serum concentrations has been defined by careful clinical studies (Levy, 1965). Paradoxically, recognition of the clinical value of knowing serum concentrations of potent drugs must not lend to their uncritical use: *therapeutic decisions should never be based solely on the drug concentrations in serum.* Drug level determinations cannot substitute for medical judgment and must always be interpreted in the context of all clinical data (Serrano et al., 1973). The following factors should be considered in all blood level interpretations:

- The effect of a given drug concentration at its site of action may be altered by many physiologic factors.
- Prolonged administration of certain drugs can result in the development of tolerance, so that higher concentrations are required for therapeutic effects.
- The therapeutic and serum toxic concentration ranges of a drug may be altered when other drugs with synergistic or antagonistic effects are concomitantly administered.
- The effective range of serum drug concentrations may differ with the disease entity.
- Serum drug concentrations can be interpreted fully only if the time elapsed since the last dose is known, and there is an understanding of steady-state plasma levels and half-lives of various drugs (Koelle, 1970).
- Protein binding of the drug should be considered (Koelle, 1970).
- Metabolic transformation of some drugs does not render them inactive; metabolites may evoke the activity of the administered drug.

An effective therapeutic regimen or antidotal measure in case of acute or chronic poisoning, requires knowledge of the relationship between the concentration of the therapeutic agent and the response of the patient at cellular and sub-cellular levels. In addition, a detailed comprehension of the factors governing the absorption, distribution, binding, biotransformation, and elimination of drugs is most essential (Figure 1).

2. Pharmacologic Basis for Monitoring Drug Levels

For an active drug molecule to be therapeutically effective it must reach the site of its intended pharmacologic activity at a sufficient rate and in sufficient amounts so that an effective concentration can be achieved. While our understanding in recent years has greatly increased regarding the mechanisms of action of most drug compounds, it is still conventional as well as a useful principle to think of a therapeutic agent as interacting with some receptor site resulting in a given pharmacologic response (Ariens et al., 1964; Paton, 1961). Feldman (1974) diagrammatically represented this interaction by the use of the following equation:

$$\text{Drug} + \text{Receptor} \rightleftharpoons \text{Drug-Receptor Complex} \rightarrow \text{Response}$$

Furthermore, the concentration of a drug at the receptor site under the conditions found *in vivo* is a function of the pharmacokinetic processes of absorption, distribution, metabolism, and excretion; such information is necessary for proper interpretation of monitoring therapeutic drug levels in plasma and serum.

The great majority of drugs appear to exert their theraputic effects after forming reversible bonds with tissue molecules or receptors. One example illustrative of the factors cited above is that of valproic acid or valproate. This is a relatively new anti-epileptic drug which has been utilized in Europe for the past ten years and has proven to be a very effective agent in the treatment of absence seizures and/or as an adjunctive agent in the treatment of generalized seizures. It is not particularly effective in the treatment of complex partial (temporal lobe) seizures.

Therapeutic monitoring of valproic acid becomes especially critical in the light of the many problems directly related to drug interactions with other antiepileptic drugs which occur following the administration of valproate.

Since this drug is 95% protein-bound, it displaces phenytoin (DPH) from its protein-binding sites. Consequently, following initial valproate therapy, patients may show a rapid decline in serum phenytoin levels. In contrast, there is a marked rise in serum phenobarbital concentrations over a period of approximately three weeks in patients receiving valproate and either phenobarbital or primidone, perhaps attributed to greater urine acidity in patients on valproate therapy.

The efficacy of biological action of drugs tends to be proportionate to drug concentrations in the vicinity of tissue receptor sites. As an example, anticonvulsant drug molecules in cerebral extracellular fluid are in a dynamic equilibrium with drug molecules in plasma. (Figure 2). Therefore, the anticonvulsant drug concentration in plasma water is a measure of anticonvulsant concentration in the brain, and thus provides a measure of antiepileptic effect. If an anticonvulsant drug in plasma is in part bound to plasma proteins, as is the case with valproic acid or phenytoin, there will be further dynamic equilibrium between the drug bound to protein, and the drug free in plasma water. Hence, the more simple measurement of drug concentration in whole plasma also provides a measure of drug concentration in the brain, and an indication of potential anticonvulsant effect. It is therefore consistent with the finding that the plasma level of the anticonvulsant is a better guide to its antiepileptic effect than the drug dose itself.

One of the more perplexing of the problems one soon discovers in theraputic drug monitoring, is one of terminology, generic vs. brand drug names, and their synonyms. While we believe that all drug references should be directed towards use of generic names, the use of brand names is still widely practiced, especially in hospitals and clinics. To this end many of our tables use the generic name as the prime source word, and Tables 1 and 2 are to be used for cross-referencing where needed.

The sources that have been used as prime source material for the drug listings in Tables 1 and 2 are Lewis (1977), Pennsylvania Bull. (1978), Goodman and Gilman (1975), Physicians Desk Reference (1978).

While many factors may effect the need for monitoring drug action, it is useful to remember that plasma levels that relate directly to pharmacologic or toxic effects are the most useful to be measured. Even when this relationship exists, the pharmacologic effect may be easy to assess more directly making a knowledge of the plasma levels totally unnecessary. This is particularly applicable to the following classes of drug compounds: diuretics, hypoglycemic agents, anti-hypertensives, anti-coagulants, analgesics and (with the possible exception of salicylates and acetaminophen) certain sedatives and hypnotics; uricosuric agents, hypolipidemics and most antimicrobial agents (with the exception of the aminoglycosides and other drugs with a narrow therapeutic index). Other indications that are generally useful for determining whether drug plasma levels should be monitored are: the prophylatic use of a drug, the presence of a narrow therapeutic range, the possible confusion between the toxic drug effect and a disease process, when oral dosages may be difficult to relate to plasma levels because of poor intestinal absorption, a drug giving zero order kinetic action, or first-pass metabolism, when tolerance is suspected (particularly true in the case of barbiturates and many of the sedatives), when prognosis and management are related to blood level after acute overdosage (a specific example in this case would be acetaminophen), when noncompliance is suspected, when the patient is suspected of drug overdosage or abuse, and when drug interaction is suspected. As an aid to the clinician and other professional people utilizing this compendium, we have arranged in tabular from the classes of compounds, both by pharmacological class and by alpha generic listing, of the various drugs presently capable of being monitored and that meet the above criteria (Tables 3 and 4). As new drugs are introduced, this list is surely to expand and physicians should be aware that many of the new compounds may require monitoring if the above criteria are applicable.

Many disease states require drug treatment over a prolonged period of time. In practice, almost all monitoring of psychotropic agents is done with

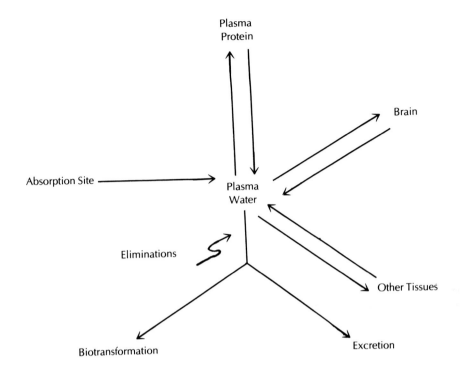

FIGURE 2. Schema of Drug Disposition in the Body
Reprinted with permission from Dr. M.J. Eadie: Clinical Pharmacokinetics, 1:52-66 (1976) and the ADIS Press.

the patient presumably in a steady state as regards intake and output of his drug. Only when treating acute crises is the monitoring of plasma drug levels done when the patient is not in the steady state.

Figure 3 presents idealized graphic representation as examples of various dose response curves and purports to give some of the generalized terminology used to depict plasma and/or blood drug levels. While these are idealized curves, one will readily see the overlapping of the therapeutic range with appropriate pharmacologic response. One can readily observe that those compounds with narrow therapeutic ranges are more likely candidates for drug monitoring than those with a wide therapeutic range and little overlapping of the toxic reactions. It is also interesting to note that patients under standardized dosages may demonstrate either a pharmacologic or a toxic reaction to this standardized dose of a particular drug compound.

The rapid growth of the practice of monitoring plasma drug levels bears witness to the practical usefulness of the procedure. However, relatively little information has been published demonstrating in statistical terms the "real" benefits to be derived from therapeutic monitoring. The monitoring of plasma drug levels are useful in many cases of possible drug overdosage, particularly when the manifestations of overdosage are unusual so that the clinical diagnosis is uncertain.

During the past several years, clinical experience has revealed that the rates of absorption, distribution, plasma and cellular binding, metabolism, and excretion of various drugs demonstrated great variability in patients. At a time when a patient may receive as many as six or more prescribed medications and be self-medicating with still others, the stage is set for adverse drug reactions. One way to avoid overdosage is to prescribe a regimen whenever possible not on the basis of body weight, but according to plasma or serum levels, especially when dealing with drugs of high potency but narrow margins of safety. This practice is particularly pertinent in patients with gastrointestinal, cardiovascular, hepatic, renal diseases or genetic abnormalities, situations in which the anticipated relation between the usual recommended dose and the actual blood level may not follow predicted values.

Bearing the above problems in mind and understanding that any recommended standard dosage can only provide guidelines for appropriate drug therapy, Table No. 5 (Standard Adult Dosages) lists the recommended dosages for those compounds which have proven amenable to drug monitoring. These data have been compiled from various sources on drug therapy and are cited to illustrate the relationship between the amount of drug administered and the measurable plasma or serum levels. In practice, these results may be greatly modified depending on the physiological, pathological, or pharmacological state of the patient; this is particularly true in the pediatric and the elderly patient and in those cases where combined drug administration is the regimen of choice.

FIGURE 3. A. **Dose - Response.** A frequency distribution curve, demonstrating the dose of an "idealized" drug required to produce specific pharmacologic and toxic responses of a specified intensity in 50% of individuals. Note that the therapeutic range demonstrates marked population variation even though the maximum pharmacologic and maximum toxicological reactions differ by a wide margin. While this "idealized" drug is demonstrated by its most prominent effects, such graphic representation should not obscure the fact that no drug produces only a single effect. In theory, the therapeutic range should be defined as the ratio between the minimum toxic dose and the maximum pharmacologic effective dose, but since assays cannot be made with accuracy in the human population, the therapeutic range (index) is defined as the ratio between the median toxic dose and the median effective dose. It is important to note that a number of individuals will experience some type of toxic symptomatology within the given therapeutic range, and that toxic reactions are directly dose dependent.

B. **Biomodal Dose - Response.** A frequency distribution curve of an "idealized" drug demonstrating primary dose response but within a given population secondary response distribution characteristics. Examples of such unusual drug response may have a hereditary basis. When such responses take the form of extremely high and low sensitivity to an ordinary effective dose, such responses are termed as 'idiosyncratic.' An example of such a response is the slow metabolism of isoniazid. Isoniazid is metabolized by N-acetylation and, to a lesser extent by hydrolysis. In a population sample, a biomodal distribution of response was found after administration of this drug, and it was in fact demonstrated that 52.2 percent of the group metabolized the drug slowly. When isoniazid is given to slow inactivators, it can accumulate to toxic levels and can result in serious neuropathies. This serves only as a single example to illustrate the large range of drug dose-response capacity in a population, and is seen more frequently the more widely serum drug levels are monitored.

C. **Blood Levels-Response Data.** An extension of Figure 3B demonstrating how serum levels can parallel pharmacologic and toxic responses and that such measurements can provide useful data to the physician to eliminate many of the toxic effects with proper dose adjustments based on clinical observations and serum drug concentration determinations.

FIGURE 3[1]

GRAPHIC EXAMPLES OF "IDEALIZED" DOSE-RESPONSE CURVES

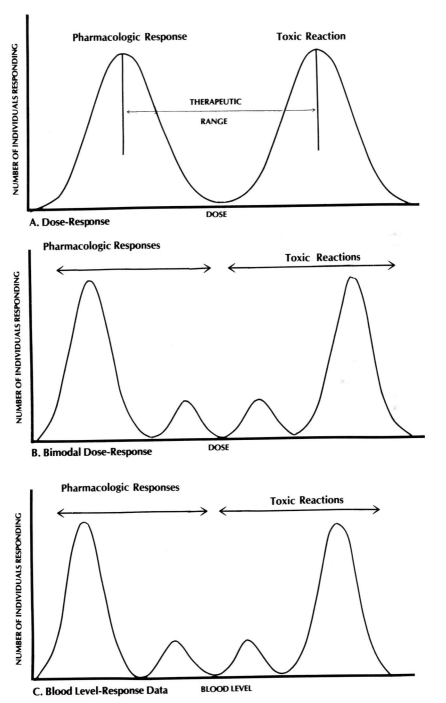

[1]Reprinted with permission from Dr. Bernard E. Cabana (J. of Pharmacokinetics and Biopharmaceuticals, Vol. 3, No. 2, 1975) and The Plenum Publishing Company, New York City, New York

TABLE 1. Brand-Generic Drug Listing

Brand Name	Generic Name	Brand Name	Generic Name
Adapin	Doxepin	Combid	Prochlorperazine
Aerolate	Theophylline	Compazine	Prochlorperazine
Airet	Dyphylline	Congespirin	Aspirin
Alurate	Aprobarbital	Cope	Aspirin
Amesec	Amobarbital	Coricidin Tablets	Aspirin
Amikin	Amikacin	Dalmane	Flurazepam
Amytal	Amobarbital	Darvocet-N	Propoxyphene
Anestacon	Lidocaine	Darvon	Propoxyphene
Antrocol	Phenobarbital	Delcobese	Amphetamine
Anturane	Sulfinpyrazone	Demerol	Meperidine
Anuphen	Acetaminophen	Depakene	Valproic Acid
APAP Capsules	Acetaminophen	Deprol	Meprobamate
Apaprin	Acetaminophen	Dexamyl	Amobarbital
A.P.B.	Phenobarbital	Dibron	Theophylline
A.P.C.	Aspirin	Dicumarol	Coumarin
A-poxide	Chlordiazepoxide	Dilantin	Phenytoin
Arco-Lase Plua	Phenobarbital	Dilor	Dyphylline
Arthralgen	Acetaminophen	Dimethadione	Dimethadione
Ascodeen-30	Aspirin	Dolophine	Methadone
Ascriptin	Aspirin	Donphen	Phenobarbital
AVC	Sulfanilamide	Doriden	Glutethimide
Aventyl	Nortriptyline	Dularin	Acetaminophen
Azene	Clorazepate	Ectasule	Amobarbital
Azotrex	Sulfamethizole	Elavil	Amitriptyline
Bactrim	Sulfamethoxazole	Elixicon	Theophylline
Bancap	Acetaminophen	Elixodyne	Acetaminophen
Bayer Aspirin	Aspirin	Elixophyllin	Theophylline
Belap	Phenobarbital	Eme-Nil	Pentobarbital
Benzedrine	Amphetamine	Emesert	Pentobarbital
Bio-Pap	Acetaminophen	Emfaseem	Dyphylline
Biphetamine	Amphetamine	Empirin	Aspirin
Bronchodid Duracap	Theophylline	Empracet	Acetaminophen
Bronkodyl	Theophylline	Emprazil	Aspirin
Bronkotabs	Theophylline	Endep	Amitriptyline
Buff-A-Comp	Aspirin	Equagestic	Aspirin
Buffadyne	Aspirin	Equanil	Meprobamate
Bufferin	Aspirin	Eskabarb	Phenobarbital
Cama Inlay - Tabs	Aspirin	Eskalith	Lithium
Capital	Acetaminophen	Eskatrol	Prochlorperazine
Cardilate-P	Phenobarbital	Etrafon	Amitriptyline
Cardioquin	Quinidine	Excedrin	Aspirin
Celontin	Methsuximide	Fetamin	Amphetamine
Cetapap	Acetaminophen	Fiorinal	Aspirin
Clonopin	Clonazepam	Gantanol	Sulfamethoxazole

TABLE 1. (cont.)

Brand Name	Generic Name	Brand Name	Generic Name
Gantrisin	Sulfisoxazole	Obetrol	Amphetamine
Garamycin	Gentamicin	Orinase	Tolbutamide
Gaysal	Phenobarbital	Oxoids	Phenobarbital
Gustase-Plus	Phenobarbital	Pabirin	Aspirin
Haldol	Haloperidol	Pamelor	Nortriptyline
Hylate	Theophylline	Pamine PB	Phenobarbital
Imavate	Imipramine	Panalgesic	Aspirin
Inderal	Propranolol	Panwarfin	Warfarin
Indocin	Indomethacin	Paradione	Paramethadione
INH	Isoniazid	Parest	Methaqualone
Janimine	Imipramine	Pathibamate	Meprobamate
Lanoxin	Digoxin	Pedraminophen No. 3	Acetaminophen
Librax	Chlordiazepoxide	Peganone	Ethotoin
Libritabs	Chlordiazepoxide	Permitil	Fluphenazine
Librium	Chlordiazepoxide	Persistin	Aspirin
Lidosporin	Lidocaine	Pertofrane	Desipramine
Lithane	Lithium	Phazyme-PB	Phenobarbital
Lithonate	Lithium	Phenaphen	Acetaminophen
Lithotabs	Lithium	Phenurone	Phenacemide
LTA II Kit	Lidocaine	Placidyl	Ethchlorvynol
Lufyllin-EPG	Dyphylline	PMB-200	Meprobamate
Marax	Theophylline	PMB-400	Meprobamate
Matropinal	Pentobarbital	Presamine	Imipramine
Measurin	Aspirin	Prolixin	Fluphenazine
Mebaral	Mephobarbital	Pronestyl	Procainamide
Mellaril	Thioridazine	Proval #3	Phenobarbital
Menrium	Chlordiazepoxide	Quaalude	Methaqualone
Meprospan	Meprobamate	Quadrinal	Theophylline
Mesantoin	Mephenytoin	Quibron	Theophylline
Methotrexate	Methotrexate	Quinaglute	Quinidine
Microsul	Sulfamethizole	Quinidex	Quinidine
Milontin	Phensuximide	Quinora	Quinidine
Milpath	Meprobamate	Rela	Carisoprodol
Miltown	Meprobamate	Rhinex	Aspirin
Monacet	Aspirin	Rifamate	Isoniazid
Mudrane	Theophylline	Rimactazid	Isoniazid
Mysoline	Primidone	Robaxisal	Aspirin
Nebcin	Tobramycin	Septra	Sulfamethoxazole
Nembutal	Pentobarbital	Serax	Oxazepam
Neothylline	Dyphylline	Sinequan	Doxepin
Nipride	Sodium Nitroprusside	SK-APAP	Acetaminophen
Norgesic	Aspirin	SK-Bamate	Meprobamate
Norpace	Disopyramide	SK-Digoxin	Digoxin
Norpramin	Desipramine	SK-Lygen	Chlordiazepoxide
Nydrazid	Isoniazid	SK-Phenobarbital	Phenobarbital
		SK-Pramine	Imipramine

TABLE 1. (cont.)

Brand Name	Generic Name	Brand Name	Generic Name
SK-Quinidine	Quinidine	Theophyl-225	Theophylline
SK-65	Aspirin	Theospan	Theophylline
SK-65 APAP	Propoxyphene	Thiosulfil	Sulfamethizole
SK-Soxazole	Sulfisoxazole	Thorazine	Chlorpromazine
Slo-Phyllin	Theophylline	Tofranil	Imipramine
Solfoton	Phenobarbital	Tolectin	Tolmetin
Solganal	Aurothioglucose	Tranxene	Clorazepate
Soma	Carisoprodol	Triavil	Amitriptyline
Somophyllin	Theophylline	Triaminicin	Aspirin
Sopor	Methaqualone	Tridione	Trimethadione
Stanol	Acetaminophen	Tuinal	Amobarbital
Suladyne	Sulfadiazine	Ty-A-Pul	Acetaminophen
Sulfamal	Sulfanilamide	Tylenol	Acetaminophen
Sultrin	Sulfacetamide	Unigesic-A	Propoxyphene
Supac	Aspirin	Vagitrol	Sulfanilamide
Synalgos	Aspirin	Valadol	Acetaminophen
Synophylate	Theophylline	Valium	Diazepam
Tapar	Acetaminophen	Valpin 50-PB	Phenobarbital
Tedral	Theophylline	Vanquish	Aspirin
Tegretol	Carbamazepine	Verequad	Phenobarbital
Theda-T	Amitriptyline	Vesprin	Triflupromazine
Theobid	Theophylline	Vivactil	Protriptyline
Theokin	Theophylline	Xylocaine	Lidocaine
Theolair	Theophylline	Zarontin	Ethosuximide
Theo-Organidin	Theophylline		

TABLE 2. Generic-Brand Drug Listing

Generic Name	Brand Name	Generic Name	Brand Name
Acetaminophen	Anuphen	Aspirin *(cont.)*	Cope
	APAP Capsules		Coricidin Tablets
	Apaprin		Empirin
	Arthralgen		Emprazil
	Bancap		Equagestic
	Bio-Pap		Excedrin
	Capital		Fiorinal
	Cetapap		Measurin
	Dularin		Monacet
	Elixodyne		Norgesic
	Empracet		Pabirin
	Pedraminophen No. 3		Panalgesic
	Phenaphen		Persistin
	Sk-APAP		Rhinex
	Stanol		Robaxisal
	Tapar		SK-65
	Ty-A-Pul		Supac
	Tylenol		Synalgos
	Valadol		Triaminicin
Amikacin	Amiken		Vanquish
Amitriptyline	Elavil	Carbamazepine	Tegretol
	Endep	Carisoprodol	Rela
	Etrafon		Soma
	Theda-T	Chlordiazepoxide	A-poxide
	Triavil		Librax
Amobarbital	Amesec		Libritabs
	Amytal		Librium
	Dexamyl		Menrium
	Ectasule		SK-Lygen
	Tuinal	Chlorpromazine	Thorazine
Amphetamine	Benzedrine	Clonazepam	Clonopin
	Biphetamine	Clorazepate	Azene
	Delcobese		Tranxene
	Fetamin	Coumarin	Dicumarol
	Obetrol	Desipramine	Norpramin
Aprobarbital	Alurate		Pertofrane
Aspirin	APC	Diazepam	Valium
(Acetylsalicylic acid)	Ascodeen-30	Dimethadione	Dimethadione
	Ascriptin	Digoxin	Lanoxin
	Bayer Aspirin		SK-Digoxin
	Buff-A-Comp	Disopyramide	Norpace
	Buffadyne	Doxepin	Adapin
	Bufferin		Sinequan
	Cama Inlay-Tabs	Dyphylline	Airet
	Congespirin		

TABLE 2. (cont.)

Generic Name	Brand Name	Generic Name	Brand Name
Dyphylline *(cont.)*	Dilor	Methadone	Dolophine
	Emfaseem	Methaqualone	Parest
	Lufyllin-EPG		Quaalude
	Neothylline		Sopor
Ethchlorvynol	Placidyl	Methotrexate	Methotrexate
Ethosuximide	Zarontin	Methsuximide	Celontin
Ethotoin	Peganone	Nortriptyline	Aventyl
Fluphenazine	Permitil		Pamelor
	Prolixin	Oxazepam	Serax
Flurazepam	Dalmane	Paramethadione	Paradione
Gentamicin	Garamycin	Pentobarbital	Eme-Nil
Glutethimide	Doriden		Emesert
Gold Salts			Matropinal
(Aurothioglucose)	Solganal		Nembutal
Haloperidol	Haldol		
Imipramine	Imavate	Phenacemide	Phenurone
	Janimine	Phenobarbital	A.P.B.
	Presamine		Antrocol
	SK-Pramine		Arco-Lase Plus
	Tofranil		Belap
Indomethacin	Indocin		Cardilate-P
Isoniazid	INH		Donphen
	Nydrazid		Eskabarb
	Rifamate		Gaysal
	Rimactazid		Gustase-Plus
Lidocaine	Anestacon		Oxoids
	Lidosporin		Pamine PB
	LTA II Kit		Phazyme-PB
	Xylocaine		Proval #3
Lithium	Eskalith		SK-Phenobarbital
	Lithane		Solfoton
	Lithonate		Valpin 50-PB
	Lithotabs		Verequad
Meperidine	Demerol	Phensuximide	Milontin
Mephenytoin	Mesantoin	Phenytoin	Dilantin
Mephobarbital	Mebaral	Primidone	Mysoline
Meprobamate	Deprol	Procainamide	Pronestyl
	Equanil	Prochlorperazine	Combid
	Meprospan		Compazine
	Milpath		Eskatrol
	Miltown	Propoxyphene	Darvocet-N
	PMB-200		Darvon
	PMB-400		SK-65 APAP
	Pathibamate		Unigesic-A
	SK-Bamate	Propranolol	Inderal

TABLE 2. (cont.)

Generic Name	Brand Name	Generic Name	Brand Name
Protriptyline	Vivactil	Theophylline (cont.)	Elixicon
Quinidine	Cardioquin		Elixophyllin
	Quinaglute		Hylate
	Quinidex		Marax
	Quinora		Mudrane
	SK-Quinidine		Quadrinal
Sodium Nitroprusside	Nipride		Quibron
Sulfacetamide	Sultrin		Slo-Phyllin
Sulfadiazine	Suladyne		Somophyllin
Sulfamethizole	Azotrex		Synophylate
	Microsul		Tedral
	Thiosulfil		Theobid
Sulfamethoxazole	Bactrim		Theokin
	Gantanol		Theolair
	Septra		Theo-Organidin
Sulfanilamide	AVC		Theophyl-225
	Sulfamal		Theospan
	Vagitrol	Thioridazine	Mellaril
Sulfathiazole	Sultrin	Tobramycin	Nebcin
Sulfinpyrazone	Anturane	Tolbutamide	Orinase
Sulfisoxazole	Gantrisin	Tolmetin	Tolectin
	SK-Soxazole	Triflupromazine	Vesprin
Theophylline	Aerolate	Trimethadione	Tridione
	Bronchodid Duracap	Valproic Acid	Depakene
	Bronkodyl	Warfarin	Panwarfin
	Bronkotabs		
	Dibron		

TABLE 3. Pharmacologic Classes of Selected Drug Compounds Ideally Suited for Therapeutic Blood Monitoring

Antibiotics

Amikacin
Chloramphenicol
Gentamicin
Isoniazid
Tobramycin

Antiarrhythmics

Digoxin
Disopyramide
Lidocaine
Procainamide
Propranolol
Quinidine

Anorexics

Chlordiazepoxide
Clorazepate
Diazepam
Oxazepam

Analgesics

Acetaminophen
Salicylates

Tranquilizers

Chlordiazepoxide
Chlorpromazine
Diazepam
Flurazepam
Haloperidol
Thioridazine

Bronchodilators

Dyphylline
Theophylline

Sedatives

Glutethimide
Phenobarbital

Antidepressants

Amitriptyline
Desipramine
Doxepin
Imipramine
Lithium
Nortriptyline
Protriptyline

Anticonvulsants

Carbamazepine
Clonazepam
Diazepam
Dimethadione
Ethosuximide
Ethotoin
Mephobarbital
Mephenytoin
Methsuximide
Paramethadione
Phenobarbital
Phensuximide
Phenytoin
Primidone
Trimethadione
Valproate, Sodium

β-Adrenergic Blocking

Propranolol

Antidiabetic

Tolbutamide

Antiarthritics

Gold Salts
Salicylates

TABLE 4. Generic Listing of Selected Drug Compounds Ideally Suited for Therapeutic Blood Monitoring

Acetaminophen	Isoniazid
Amikacin	Lidocaine
Amitriptyline	Lithium
Carbamazepine	Mephobarbital
Chloramphenicol	Mephenytoin
Chloridiazepoxide	Methsuximide
Chlorpromazine	Methotrexate
Clonazepam	Nortriptyline
Clorazepate	Paramethadione
Desipramine	Phenobarbital
Diazepam	Phensuximide
Digoxin	Phenytoin
Dimethadione	Primidone
Disopyramide	Procainamide
Doxepin	Propranolol
Dyphylline	Protriptyline
Ethosuximide	Quinidine
Ethotoin	Salicylates
Flurazepam	Theophylline
Gentamicin	Thioridazine
Glutethimide	Tobramycin
Gold salts	Tolbutamide
Haloperidol	Trimethadione
Imipramine	Valproate, sodium

TABLE 5. STANDARD ADULT DOSAGE TABLE[1]

Generic Name	Standard Daily Dosage	Remarks
Acetaminophen	Adult: 0.3-0.6 gm	Every 4-6 hours
	Pediatric: 60 mg/kg/day	Given in 4-6 doses
Amikacin	Adult: 0.5 gm IM (15 mg/kg/day)	Every 6-12 hours
	Pediatric: 10-20 mg/kg/day (IM)	Every 12 hours
		Dosages only applicable if renal
		clearance is 100-200 ml/min.
Amitriptyline	25 mg 3 times/day	Maximum daily dose: 150 mg
		May require
		3-30 days of drug therapy
Amobarbital	Hypnotic: 100-200 ng	Single dose
	Sedative: 15-30 mg	3-4 times daily
Amphetamine	5 mg	3 times daily before meals
		(15 mg single dose equally
		effective)
Aprobarbital	Sedative: 40 mg	3 times daily
	Mild insomnia: 40-80 mg	At bedtime
	Pronounced insomnia: 80-160 mg	At bedtime
	Antipyretic-analgesic:	
Aspirin	Adult: 0.3-1 gm (10-15 mg/kg)	Every 4-6 hours
(Acetylsalicylic Acid)	Pediatric: 60 mg/kg/day	Given in 4-6 doses
	Anti-inflammatory:	
	Adults: 3-6 g/day	In 4-6 doses
	Children: 25 mg/kg/day	For 1-2 days)
	18 mg/kg/day	For 7-10 days) 4-6 hour doses
	14 mg/kg/day	As necessary)
Carbamazepine	Initial dose: 400 mg/day	4 doses (orally)
	Maintenance dose: 800-1200 mg/day	4 doses (orally)
	(10-20 mg/kg)	
Carisoprodol	350 mg	3 times daily and at bedtime
Chlordiazepoxide	Sedative: 10-20 mg	3-4 times daily
Chlorpromazine	100-600 mg	Daily as single bedtime dose
		Doses of 100-200 mg IV or/IM
		may be required in some psy-
		chotic states
Clonazepam	Initial dose: 0.02 mg/kg/day	Orally
	Maintenance dose: Increase dosage	Orally
	by 0.015 mg/kg/day every 3-4 days	
	to maximum of 0.3 mg/kg/day	
Clorazepate	Sedative: 7.5 mg	3-4 times daily
Coumarin	First day: 200-400 mg	Orally
(Bishydroxycoumarin)	Second day: 100-200 mg	
	Maintenance dose: 25-150 mg	
Desipramine	25 mg 3 times/day	Maximum daily dose: 200 mg
Diazepam	Sedative: 5 mg	3-4 times daily
	Anxiety: 5-10 mg	Daily

[1]Sources for most of the data contained in Table 5 have been taken from Goldstein et al. (1974), Meyers et al. (1976), Opie (1980a, 1980b, 1980c), Bochner (1978), Physicians' Desk Reference (1980), AACC (1980), Bleyer (1978).

TABLE 5. (cont'd)

Generic Name	Standard Daily Dosage	Remarks

Digoxin	Digitalizing dose:
	    Oral: 1-1.5 mg (10-15 mg/kg)
	    IV: 0.5-1.0 mg	

	Maintenance dose: 0.25-0.75 mg (3-5 mg/kg)	Orally

	Children dosage (Oral):
	    Premature/newborn:10-12.5 mg/kg/day
	    1 month-1 year: 20-25 mg/kg/day
	    1 year-2 year: 16-20 mg/kg/day
	    2-12 years: 10-15 mg/kg/day	

Digitoxin	Digitalizing dose: Oral: 1.2-1.5 mg (10 mg/kg)	IV: 1.2 mg
	Maintenance dose: 0.1-0.2 mg (1.5 mg/kg)	Orally
Disopyramide	Ventricular arrhythmias: IV: 2 mg/kg over 5 min.	Maximum 150 mg and up to 300 mg in first hour (0.4 mg/kg)
	Oral: 300 mg loading dose, then 100-150 mg	Every 6 hours - maximum 200 mg every 6 hours

	Supraventricular arrhythmias
	    IV: 2 mg/kg over 5 min. Repeat
	        up to 300 mg/hour	

Doxepin	25 mg 3 times/day	Maximum daily dose: 300 mg
Dyphylline	Orally: 15 mg/kg IM: 500 mg	Every 6 hours Repeated as necessary
Ethchlorvynol	Hypnotic: 500 mg Sedative: 100-200 mg	Orally 3-4 times daily; not recommended for continuous sedation
Ethosuximide	250-500 mg (5 mg/kg)	2 times/day
Ethotoin	0.5-1 gm	2-3 times/day
Fluphenazine	2 mg	Daily (oral)
Flurazepam	Hypnotic: 15-30 mg	
Gentamicin	Adult: 102 mg/kg Pediatric: 1-3 mg/kg	Every 8 hours Dosages only applicable if renal clearance is 100-120 ml/min
Gitalin (Gitaligin)	Digitalizing dose: Oral: 5 mg	
	Maintenance dose: 0.5 mg	Orally
Glutethimide	Hypnotic: 500 mg Sedative: 125-250 mg	Single dose 3-4 times daily; not recommended for continuous sedation

Gold Salts
(Aurothio Glucose)
(Gold Sodium Thioglucose)
	Dosage regimen (IM):
	    1st week: 10 mg
	    2nd week: 25 mg
	    3rd week: 25 mg
	    50 mg weekly for total dose of 750 mg
		Once remission occurs the following dosage should be followed:
		4 doses of 50 mg at 2 week interval; 4 doses of 50 mg at 3 week interval; every month - 50 mg for 1 year

TABLE 5. (cont'd)

Generic Name	Standard Daily Dosage	Remarks
Haloperidol	0.5-30 mg	Must be adjusted clinically to patient's need; doses up to 1000 mg/day have been used. Incidence of side effects increases with doses 30 mg/day
Imipramine	25 mg 3 times daily	Maximum daily dose: 200 mg Patients who have received MAOI should not receive imipramine within 2 weeks of stopping MAOI
Indomethacin	25-50 mg	3 times daily In acute gout 200-400 mg/day for 2-3 days may be used
Isoniazid	Initial dosage: Adults: 8-10 mg/kg/day Pediatric: 20 mg/kg/day Post Initial Improvement: Adults: 5-7 mg/kg/day Pediatric: 10 mg/kg/day	Orally Orally Orally Orally Children converting from tuberculin negative to positive skin results: 5-10 mg/kg/day (max. 300 mg/day) for 1 year as prophylaxis for meningitis (not recommended for patients over 35 yrs.)
Lidocaine	Initial dosages: IV: 1-2 mg/kg in 30 seconds Continuous infusion: IV: 1-3 mg/minute	To maintain clinical effect as needed
Lithium	Initial dosage: 600 mg 3 times/day Maintenance dosage: 300 mg 3 times/day (15-20 mg/kg)	Serum level should not exceed 1.5 mEq/liter Dosage should give serum Li levels of 0.5-1.0 mEq/L; single dose may be satisfactory when steady state revealed
Meperidine	Subcut dosage: 75-150 mg (IM) Oral dosage: 75-100 mg (1.0-1.5 mg/kg)	Recommended single dose
Mephenytoin	100-300 mg	2 times/day
Mephobarbital	200-400 mg/day	Divided doses
Mephrobamate	Sedative: 400 mg	Not recommended for continuous sedation
Methadone	Subcut dosage: 5 mg (SC) Oral dosage: 5 mg	Recommended single dose

TABLE 5. (cont'd)

Generic Name	Standard Daily Dosage	Remarks
Methaqualone	Hypnotic: 150-300 mg	
Methotrexate	Adult: variable	
	Pediatric: variable	

A common protocol for using methotrexate as an anti-tumor agent calls for massive doses of the drug, followed by a rescue from the cytotoxic effects by administration of 5-formyl-tetrahydrofolic acid (citrovorum factor). Such high dose protocols, require the monitoring of serum methotrexate levels, to assess potential drug cytotoxicity. Additional clinical determination that may prove useful include urinary flow, urine pH, serum creatinine and creatinine clearance.

There is also a direct and predictable relationship in man between the dosage administered and the plasma levels. To achieve a desired initial plasma level, the following formula may be useful (Bleyer, 1978).

$$\text{Priming Dose (mg/m}^2) = (1.5 \times 10^7)(MTX_p)$$

where MTX_p is the desired plasma level in moles/L. To maintain the plasma concentration at a given level, the following formula may be used provided renal function is normal:

$$\text{Infusion Dose (mg/m}^2/\text{hour}) = (3 \times 10^6)(MTX_p)$$

Other basic treatment regimens include conventional low dosage without citrovorum factor and intrathecal methotrexate therapy. For conversion of mg/kg to mg/m² or reverse, a ratio of 1:30 is used as a guide.

Suggested dosage guides follow:

1. Choriocarcinoma (trophoblastic): 15-30 mg daily (IM/oral) for 5 days.

2. Leukemia (lymphoblastic): Initial dose: 3.3 mg/m² daily for 4-6 weeks; After remission: 30 mg/m² twice weekly (IM/oral) or 2.5 mg/kg (IV) every 14 days.

3. Lymphomas: In Burkitt's Tumor, Stages I-II, methotrexate has produced prolonged remissions in some cases. Recommended dosage is 10 to 25 mg per day orally for 4 to 8 days. In Stage III, methotrexate is commonly given concomitantly with other antitumor agents. Treatment in all stages usually consists of several courses of the drug interposed with 7 to 10 day rest periods. Lymphosarcomas in Stage III may respond to combined drug therapy with methotrexate given in doses of 0.625 mg to 2.5 mg/kg daily. Hodgkin's Disease responds poorly to methotrexate and to most types of chemotherapy.

4. Psoriasis Chemotherapy:

(a) Weekly single oral, IM of IV dose schedule: 10-25 mg per week until adequate response is achieved. With this dosage schedule, 50 mg per week should ordinarily not be exceeded.

(b) Divided oral dose schedule: 2.5 mg at 12 hour intervals for three doses or at 8 hour intervals for four doses each week. With this dosage schedule, 30 mg per week should not be exceeded.

(c) Daily oral dose schedule: 2.5 mg daily for five days followed by at least a two day rest period. With this dosage schedule, 6.25 mg per day should not be exceeded.

Special Note: Available data suggest that schedule (c) may carry an increased risk of serious liver pathology.

Dosages in each schedule may be gradually adjusted to achieve optimal clinical response, but not to exceed the maximum stated for each schedule.

Once optimal clinical response has been achieved, each dosage schedule should be reduced to the lowest possible amount of drug and to the longest possible rest period. The use of methotrexate may permit the return to conventional topical therapy, which should be encouraged.

Methsuximide	0.3-0.6 gm	2 times/day
Nortriptyline	10 mg 3 times daily	Maximum daily dose: 100 mg
Oxazepam	Sedative: 15-30 mg	3-4 times daily
Paramethadione	300 mg	1-4 times/day

TABLE 5. (cont'd)

Generic Name	Standard Daily Dosage	Remarks
Pentobarbital	Hypnotic: 100-200 mg	Single dose
	Sedative: 30 mg	3-4 times daily; not recommended for continuous sedation
Phenacemide	1 gm (oral)	2-3 times daily
Phenobarbital	Hypnotic: 100 mg	Single dose
	Sedative: 15-30 mg	3-4 times daily
	Anticonvulsant: 100-200 mg/day (1-3 mg/kg)	May be up to 400 mg/day
Phensuximide	0.5-1 gm	2 times/day
Phenytoin	100-300 mg	1-2 times/daily
	2-6 mg/kg	
Primidone	Initial dosage: 50 mg	3 times daily
	Maintenance dosage: 250-500 mg	3 times daily, as required
Procainamide	IV: 100 mg loading dose over 2 min.; up to 20 mg/min. maintenance: 2-6 mg/min.	Maximum 1 gm in first hour
	Oral: Initial 1 gm dose; then up to 500 mg every 3 hours	Toxic effect occurs at serum levels in excess of 16 mg/L.
Prochlorperazine	Anxiety Control:	
	Oral: 5-10 mg	3 to 4 times daily
	Rectal: 25mg	Twice daily
	IM: 5-10 mg	If necessary, repeat 3-4 hours; maximum daily IM dose: 40 mg
	Adult Surgery:	
	IM: 5-10 mg	1-2 hours before induction of anesthesia; repeat once in 30 minutes if necessary.
	IV: 5-10 mg	15-30 minutes before induction of anesthesia
	IV (infusion): 20 mg/L isotomic solution	Add to IV infusion 15-30 minutes before induction of anesthesia
	Adult Psychiatry:	
	Mild: 5-10 mg (oral)	3-4 times daily
	Moderate to Severe: 10 mg	3-4 times daily
	Dosage should be increased gradually, in small increments every 2-3 days, until desired effect is achieved.	Patients have responded satisfactorily on 50-75 mg daily
	Severe Disturbances:	
	Oral: 100-150 mg	Daily
	IM: 10-20 mg	Every 2-4 hours, or as needed; more than 3-4 doses are seldom necessary.
Propoxyphene	As hydrochloride: 65 mg	Every 4 hours, as needed for pain
	As napsylate: 1000 mg	Every 4 hours, as needed for pain
Propranolol	Antiaginal/Antiarrhythimic:	
	Oral: 40-160 mg	In 2-4 divided doses. Dose may be increased to 3000 mg/day if no toxic effects.
	IV: Initial dose of 1 mg	Repeated as necessary, separate by 10-20 minutes
	Thyrotoxicosis: Higher doses may be needed	

TABLE 5. (cont'd)

Generic Name	Standard Daily Dosage	Remarks
Protriptyline	5-10 mg 3 times daily	Maximum daily dose: 60 mg
Quinidine	Conversion dosages: Oral: 1st day: 0.2 gm	Every 2 hours until toxicity, therapeutic, or 4-5 doses been given
	2nd day: 0.4 gm	Every 2 hours for 5 doses
	Subsequent days: increased to 0.6 gm	Every 2 hours for 5 doses
	IM: Same as oral dosage	
	IV: 0.8 gm in 10 ml ampules diluted with 50-100 ml 5% glucose - infused at rate of 1 ml/minute	IV route should be used in urgent situations, with frequent ECG's and blood pressure
	Maintenance (prevention) dosage: 0.2-0.4 gm (oral)	4 times daily. Reliability of sustained-release preparations has not been fully confirmed.
Sodium nitroprusside	10 μg/min (IV); up by 10 μg/min every 10 min. to 40-75 μg/min	Maximum dosage: 300 μg/min
Sulfacetamide	140-150 mg	Intravaginary at bedtime and again in morning for 7-10 days

Sulfadiazine	Initial Dosage:
	   2-4 gm (40 mg/kg)
	Maintenance Dosage:
	   0.5-1 gm (15 mg/kg)
		Every 4-6 hours

Sulfamethizole	0.5-1 gm (10 mg/kg)	In daily doses
Sulfamethoxazole	0.5-1 gm (10 mg/kg)	Given at 12 hour intervals for 8-14 days
Sulfanilamide	1.0 gm	Intravaginary 1-2 times daily, for one complete menstrual cycle. Improvement should occur in a few days
Sulfathiazole	170-175 mg	Intravaginary at bedtime and again in morning for 7-10 days
Sulfinpyrazone	Initial Dose: 100-200 mg Increase dose gradually to 400 mg	In 3 divided doses In 3 divided doses

Sulfisoxazole	Initial Dosage:
	   2-4 gm (40 mg/kg)
	Maintenance Dosage:
	   0.5-1.0 gm (15 mg/kg)
		Every 4-6 hours

Theophylline	Oral: 10-15 mg/kg/day theophylline equivalent	In 3-4 daily doses

	Aminophylline (80% theophylline):
	   Loading dose: 5-6 mg/kg IV
	   Maintenance dose: 0.9 mg/kg/hr IV
		Over 20 minutes
		Serum levels of theophylline
		should range 5-15 mg/L

Thioridazine	100 mg (oral)	Daily
Tobramycin	Adult: 1-2 mg/kg Pediatric: 1-3 mg/kg	Every 8 hours Every 8 hours (Doses only applicable if renal clearance is 100-120 ml/min.)
Tolbutamide	0.5-3.0 gm	In divided daily doses
Tolmetin	400 mg	3 times daily

TABLE 5. (cont'd)

Generic Name	Standard Daily Dosage	Remarks
Triflupromazine	30 mg (oral)	Daily
Trimethadione	300 mg	1-4 times/day
Valprioc acid (sodium valproate)	3-30 mg/kg	Average adult dosage is 1200 mg/day
Warfarin	First day: 30-50 mg	IV
	Second day: 10-15 mg	Note only warfarin of the
	Maintenance dose: 5-15 mg	prothrombin depressants may be given IV.

Table 6 (Toxic Clinical manifestations with Selected Drug Therapy) has been compiled to provide guidelines for a number of compounds that fullfill the criteria for monitoring and those toxicological symptoms that may occur with standard pharmacologic doses.

TABLE 6. Toxic clinical Manifestations with Selected Drug Therapy

Clinical Manifestation	Causal Drug(s)
DERMATOLOGICAL	
Exfoliative Dermatitis:	Penicillin
	Sulfonamides
	Barbiturates
	Mesantoin
	Phenytoin
	Phenylbutazone
	Gold Salts
	Phenothiazines
	Quinidine
Stevens-Johnson Syndrome:	Penicillin
	Sulfonamides
	Phenytoin
	Trimethadione
	Phenobarbital
	Aspirin
	Phenothiazines
	Gold Salts
	Chloramphenicol
	Carbamazepine
	Digoxin
Toxic Epidermal Necrolysis:	Phenylbutazone
	Phenytoin
	Sulfonamides
	Barbiturates
	Gold Salts

TABLE 6. (cont'd)

Clinical Manifestation	Causal Drug(s)
Furunculoid (Acne) Eruptions:	Corticosteriods Oral Contraceptives Bromides Isoniazid Haloperidol
Contact Dermatitis:	Chloramphenicol Chlorpromazine Meprobamate Neomycin Penicillin Procaine Sulfonamides
Erythema Nodosum:	Sulfonamides Bromides Salicylates Phenacetin Barbiturates Thiazides Phenytoin Trimethadione
Rashes:	May be caused by various drug compounds
Fixed Eruptions:	Phenacetin Barbiturates Sulfonamides Salicylates Phenytoin Mesantoin Trimethadione Carisoprodol Gold Salts Meprobamate Penicillin Quinidine
Photosensitive Reactions:	Sulfonamides Tolbutamide Chlorpromazine Prochlorperazine Promazine Promethazine Chlorothiazide Hydrochlorothiazide Haloperidol Chlordiazepoxide

TABLE 6. (cont'd)

Clinical Manifestation	Causal Drug(s)
Urticaria:	Ampicillin
	Penicillin
	Chloramphenicol
	Aspirin
	Barbiturates
	Morphine
	Meperidine
	Codeine
	Propoxyphene
	Bromides
	Phenytoin
	Isoniazid
	Meprobamate
Hyperpigmentation: (various varieties)	Chlorpromazine
	Phenytoin
	Gold Salts
	Chloroquine
	Salicylates
	Bromides
Alopecia:	Various cytoxic drugs. including methotrexate and 5-fluorouracil
	Trimethadione
	Heparin
Hirsutism:	Phenytoin
	Chlorpromazine
	Oral Contraceptives

HEMATOLOGICAL

Aplastic Anemia:	Methotrexate
	5-Fluorouracil
	Vin Blastine
	Chloramphenicol
	Sulfonamides
	Penicillin
	Phenylbutazone
	Aspirin
	Indomethacin
	Mephenytoin
	Trimethadione
	Phenytoin
	Primidone
	Gold Salts
	Chlorpromazine
	Promazine
	Triflupromazine
	Chlordiazepoxide
	Tolbutamide
	Chlorothiazide
	Thiocyanate
	Carbamazepine

TABLE 6. (cont'd)

Clinical Manifestation	Causal Drug(s)
Hemolytic Anemias:	Sulfanilamide
	Sulfapyridine
	Sulfisoxazole
	Quinidine
	Phenacetin
	Aspirin
	Chloramphenicol
Immune Hemolysis:	Penicillin
(positive direct coombs)	Quinidine
	Sulfonamides
	Chlorpromazine
Megaloblastic Anemia:	Methotrexate
	Trimethoprim
	Phenytoin
	Primidone
	Barbiturates
	Salicylates
	Phenylbutazone
Iron Deficiency Anemia:	Aspirin
	Isoniazid
Pure Erythrocyte Aplasia:	Chloramphenicol
	Phenytoin
	Sulfathiazole
	Phenobarbital
	Tolbutamide
Methemoglobinemia/Sulfhemo-	Phenacetin
globinemia:	Nitrates
	Nitrites
	Sulfonamides
	Chloroquine
Agranulocytosis:	Vincristine
	Phenylbutazone
	Aspirin
	Phenacetin
	Chloramephenicol
	Ampicillin
	Sulfonamides
	Chlorpromazine
	Promazine
	Prochlorperazine

TABLE 6. (cont'd)

Clinical Manifestation	Causal Drug(s)
	Tolbutamide
	Thiazides
	Phenytoin
	Trimethadione
	Ethosuximide
	Meprobamate
	Imipramine
	Desipramine
	Procainamide
	Barbiturates
	Gold Salts
Thrombocytopenia:	Phenacetin
	Aspirin
	Salicylates
	Acetaminophen
	Phenylbutazone
	Codeine
	Meperidine
	Quinidine
	Sulfonamides
	Chloramphenicol
	Isoniazid
	Phenytoin
	Barbiturates
	Meprobamate
	Prochlorperazine
	Promethazine
	Desipramine
	Thiazides
	Tolbutamide
	Mephenytoin
	Trimethadione
	Paramethadione
	Gold Salts
	Dextroamphetamine
	Digitoxin
	Carbamazepine
	Heparin
	Chloroquine
	Procaine

TABLE 6. (cont'd)

Clinical Manifestation	Causal Drug(s)

Coagulation Defects:
    Increase prothrombin time:

	Phenylbutazone
	Indomethacin
	Salicylates
	Phenytoin
	Quinidine

    Decrease prothrombin time:

	Barbiturates
	Chloral hydrate
	Glutethimide
	Meprobamate
	Halperidol
	Ethchlorvynol

Lymph Disorders:
    Pseudolymphoma syndrome:

	Phenytoin
	Mephenytoin
	Phensuximide
	Ethotoin
	Primidone

Lymph node enlargement:

	Phenylbutazone
	Meprobamate

CARDIOVASCULAR

Drug-Induced Arrhythmias:
  Sinus tachycardia:

	Anyl nitrite
	Phenothiazines

Sinus bradycardia:

	Digitalis
	Propranolol
	Phenytoin

Sinoatrial block:

	Digitalis
	Quinidine
	Salicylates

Atrial tachycardia:

	Digitalis
	Methylphenidate

Atrial flutter:

	Digitalis
	Quinidine

Atrial fibrillation:

	Digitalis
	Methylphenidate

TABLE 6. (cont'd)

Clinical Manifestation	Causal Drug(s)
Atrioventricular dissociation:	Digitalis Quinidine Procainamide Salicylates
Complete heart block:	Digitalis Propranolol
Premature ventricular contractions:	Digitalis Quinidine Procainamide
Ventricular tachycardia:	Digitalis Quinidine Procainamide Thioridazine
Ventricular fibrillation:	Digitalis Quinidine Procainamide
Hypertension:	pentazocine
Hypotension:	Hydrochlorothiazide Procainamide Phenytoin Propranolol Chlorpromazine Imipramine Amitriptyline Chloramphenicol

GASTROINTESTINAL

(Various adverse reactions, including nausea, vomiting, and diarrhea)	Various drugs including: Amitriptyline Imipramine Phenytoin Phenylbutazone Vincristine Digoxin Salicylates Indomethacin Aspirin Tolbutamide Ethanol

TABLE 6. (cont'd)

Clinical Manifestation	Causal Drug(s)
	Quinidine
	Ampicillin
	Chlorothiazide
	Pentobarsione

HEPATIC DYSFUNCTIONS

Cholestatic Jaundice:	Chlorpromazine
	Promazine
	Trifluoperazine
	Thioridazine
	Fluphenazine
	Prochloperazine
	Trimeprazine
	Chlordiazepoxide
	Meprobamate
	Imipramine
	Amitriptyline
	Desipramine
	Nortriptyline
	Oral Contraceptives
	Tolbutamide
	Sulfonamides
	Chlorathiazide
	Indomethacin
	Carbamazepine
Hepatocellular Jaundice:	Isoniazid
	Para-aminosalicylic acid
	Sulfonamides
	Penicillin
	Phenylbutazone
	Indomethacin
	Gold Salts
	Aspirin
	Mithramycin
	Chlorambucil
	Chloramphenicol
	Phenacemide
	Phenytoin
	Mephenytoin
	Ethotoin
	Trimethadione
	Phenobarbital
	Thiouracil
	Chlordiazepoxide
	Carbamazepine

TABLE 6. (cont'd)

Clinical Manifestation	Causal Drug(s)
Fibrosis or Cirrhosis:	Chlorpromazine Tolbutamide Methotrexate Chlorambucil

PULMONARY DYSFUNCTION
Asthma:	Aspirin Indomethacin Propranolol
Infiltrates or Fibrosis:	Hydrochlorothiazide Methotrexate
Mediastinal Involvement:	Phenytoin Methotrexate

ENDOCRINOLOGICAL
Hyperglycemia:	Oral Contraceptives Thiazide Diuretics Insulin Phenytoin Isoniazid Lithium Carbonate
Hypoglycemia:	Insulin Propranolol Tolbutamide Sulfonamides Phenylbutazone Salicylates Thiazide diuretics Alcohol
Galactorrhea:	Oral Contraceptives Trifluoperazine Thioridazine Haloperidol Chlordiazepoxide Imipramine Amitriptyline

RENAL DYSFUNCTIONS
Nephrotoxicity:	Gold Salts Phenacetin Salicylates Phenylbutazone Sulfonamides Streptomycin Kanamycin Gentamycin Neomycin Penicillin Ampicillin Vancomycin

TABLE 6. (cont'd)

Clinical Manifestation	Causal Drug(s)
	Cyclophosphamide Thiazide Diuretics Quinine
Nephrotic Syndrome:	Gold Salts Trimethadione Tolbutamide
Nephrogenic Diabetes Insipidus:	Lithium Carbonate
Hemorrhagic Cystitis:	Cyclophosphamide

METABOLIC DISORDERS

Electrolyte Imbalance:	Diuretics Chlorpropamide Vincristine Potassium Salts Antineoplastics Insulin
Acid-base Changes:	diuretics Acetazolamide
Fluid Imbalance:	Phenylbutazone Oral Contraceptives
Hypercalcemia:	Thiazide Diuretics
Hypocalcemia:	Mithramycin
Hyperuricemia:	Thiazide Diuretics Aspirin (low dose)
Prophyria:	Barbiturates Chlordiazepoxide Meprobamate Sulfonamides Phenytoin Tolbutamide Oral Contraceptives Alcohol

NEUROLOGICAL DISORDERS

Peripheral Neuropathies:	Digoxin Gold Salts Isoniazid Kanamycin Vancomycin Chloramphenicol Imipramine Amitriptyline Vincristine
Extrapyramidal Syndromes:	Phenothiazines Haloperidol Barbiturates

TABLE 6. (cont'd)

Clinical Manifestation	Causal Drug(s)

Seizures:	Amphetamines
	Phenothiazines
	Imipramine
	Amitriptyline
	Isoniazid
	Lidocaine
	Barbiturate withdrawal
	Ethchlorvynol withdrawal
	Glutethimide withdrawal
	Monamine oxidase inhibitors
	   combined with either
	     imipramine or anitriptyline
	Phenothiazines combined
	with piperazine

CNS Depression or Coma:	Amitriptyline Sedatives Combination Drug Regimens Salicylates Insulin Chlorpromazine Imipramine
Ataxia:	Phenytoin Isoniazid Chlordiazepoxide
Anxiety:	Amphetamines Amitriptyline Imipramine Barbiturates
Depression:	Oral contraceptives Chlordiazepoxide Diazepam
Drug-Induced Psychoses:	Oral Contraceptives Prochlorperazine Carbamazepine Isoniazid ampicillin Digoxin Barbiturate withdrawal Diazepam withdrawal

COMBINED SYSTEM REACTIONS

Fever:	Penicillin Isoniazid Amphotericin B Sulfonamides Barbiturates Phenytoin Procainamide Quinidine Salicylates

TABLE 6. (cont'd)

Clinical Manifestation	Causal Drug(s)
Systemic Lupus Erythematosus (SLE):	Procainamide Isoniazid Phenytoin Mephenytoin Primidone Trimethadione Ethosuximide Methsuximide Barbiturates Sulfonamides Quinidine Phenylbutazone Chlorpromazine Methotrimeprazine Perphenazine Promazine
Vasculitis:	Penicillin Sulfonamides Phenylbutazone Quinidine Quinine Chlorpromazine Phenytoin Gold Salts Barbiturates Procainamide Chlorothiazide Salicylates
"Serum Sickness":	Penicillins Sulfonamides Barbiturates Digitalis Phenytoin Heparin Insulin Isoniazid Phenylbutazone Procainamide Quinidine Quinine Salicylates Streptomycin
Anaphylaxis:	Penicillin Tetracyclines Sterptomycin Sulfonamides Procaine Insulin Salicylates Heparin Meprobamate Triphenylmethane (dye to determine burn depth)

TABLE 7. Correlation of Toxic Effects with Serum Drug Levels

Drug	Drug/Metabolite Measured	Serum Level, mg/liter	Toxicological Data — Clinical Findings
Acetaminophen	Same	150-3000	Circulatory collapse; confusion; low blood pressure; nausea; vomiting; jaundice; acute renal failure; liver necrosis, death. Plasma concentrations of 250 mg/liter after 4 hours post-ingestion are usually associated with hepatotoxicity. A useful index of liver necrosis is the half-life ($t_{1/2}$) at 4-12 hours post-administration—a $t_{1/2}$ greater than 4 hours suggests liver damage.
Amitriptyline	Parent compound and nortriptyline	1.0 and greater; possible genetic role in toxic levels	QRS duration > 100m sec; unconsciousness, abnormal deep tensor reflexes; respiratory depression; seizures; cardiac arrhythmia; cardiac arrest; coma. Fatalities have been reported with levels of 2 mg/liter and greater
Amobarbital	Same		Clinical Stages
		5-10	(1) Awake, competent; mildly sedated
		15-25	(2) Sedated; reflexes present; prefers sleep; does not cerebrate
		25-45	(3) Comatose; reflexes present
		45-60	(4) Comatose; areflexia
		60	(5) Comatose; circulatory and/or respiratory difficulty
			These clinical stages do not have definite limits, but blend into each other as the patient progresses from stage to stage; the concentration given represents the average range for nontolerant patients.
			The deep tendon reflexes were used as the criteria for presence or absence of reflexes; gag and cough reflexes return at approximately the same time as the deep tendon reflexes

TABLE 7. (cont'd)

Amphetamine	Same	Not fully established	Tremulousness; anxiety; awareness of heart action; dry mouth; insomnia; toxic psychosis; hypertension; tachycardia; weight loss; state of perception similar to schizophenia; auditory and visual hallucinations Deaths have been reported at levels in excess of 2 mg/liter
Aspirin (acetylsalicylic acid)	Same	> 150; dependent upon duration of poisoning and drug intake	Acute: Hyperpnea; lethargy; vomiting; tinnitus; excitability; delirium; dehydration; ecchymoses; coma; convulsions; uremia; hypoglycemia Chronic: Tinnitus; abnormal bleeding; ulcer; weight loss; skin eruptions. The following levels have been associated with specific clinical findings: Tinnitus; vertigo: > 200 mg/liter Hepatotoxicity: 200-400 mg/liter Coma; cardiovascular collapse: 400-900 mg/liter
Carbamazepine	Same	10-15 and greater	Aplastic anemia; agranulocytosis; jaundice; skin rash; hypertension; cardiac failure. Levels of greater than 9 mg/liter have been shown to produce drowsiness
Carisoprodol	Same	Greater than 50	Drowsiness; skin rashes
Chlordiazepoxide	Same	5-20	Stimulation; rage reaction; dermatitis; confusion; jaundice; agranulocytosis; convulsions
Chlorpromazine	Same	1-2	Drowiness; mild hypotension; hypothermia; tachycardia; nausea; ataxia; anorexia; coma; agranulocytosis; jaundice; skin pigmentation
Clonazepam	Same	Not Established	Possible synergism with other anticonvulsants and depressants; excitability; ataxia; dysarthria; weight gain
Clorazepate	Nordiazepam	Not fully established	Abnormal liver and kidney function tests; hypotension; skin rash
Desipramine	Same	1.5	QRS duration 100m sec; unconsciouness; seizures; cardiac arrhythmia; hypotension; cardiac arrest
Diazepam	Same	5-20	Tinnitus excitability; rage reaction; hallucinations; synergism with other depressants. Psychological dependence may occur

TABLE 7. (cont'd)

		Toxicological Data	
Drug	Drug/Metabolite Measured	Serum Level, mg/liter	Clinical Findings
Digoxin	Same	Symptoms may be observed at levels of 1.7 ng/ml and greater	Headache; vomiting; blurred vision; delirium; irregular pulse; fall of blood pressure. Digoxin exhibits a very low margin of safety, and it has been shown that hypokalemia and hypomagnesemia may potentiate toxicity
Disopyramide	Same	Not fully established, but are thought to exceed 9.0	Excessive widening of the QRS complex; worsening of congestive heart failure;hypotension; conduction disturbance; bradycardia; asystole; anti-cholinergic effects including urinary retention, dry mouth, constipation, blurred vision
Doxepin	Nordoxepin	1.6–2.5	QRS duration > 100m sec; unconsciousness; seizures; cardiac arrhythmia; hypotension; cardiac arrest
Dyphylline	Same	> 20	Concomitant therapy with sympathomimetics may induce restlessness; insomnia, cardiac arrhythmias; anorexia, nausea, occasional vomiting; agitated maniacal behavior and extreme thirst; delirium; convulsions; hyperthermia; vasomotor collapse
Ethchlorvynol	Same	Greater than 20	Hypothermia; bradycardia; hypotension; drowsiness; pungent aromatic breath; coma
Ethosuximide	Same	100–200	Periorbital edema; proteinuria; hepatic dysfunction; bone marrow aplasia; delayed coma; a syndrome similar to systemic lupus erythematosus (SLE) has been observed
Ethotoin	Same	Not fully established	Nausea; vomiting
Fluphenazine	Same	Not established	Extrapyramidal symptoms including pseudo-Parkinsonism, dystonia, dyskinesia, akathisis, and hyperreflexia; persistent tardive dyskinesia; hypertension; nausea; loss of appetite; perpheral edema; skin disorders; agranulocytosis; cholestatic jaundice; lupus-like syndrome (SLE); altered CNS proteins

TABLE 7. (cont'd)

Drug	Active compound	Level	Toxic effects
Flurazepam	Parent compound plus N-desalkyl-flurazepam metabolite	Greater than 0.2	Somnolence; confusion; coma. Death has occurred at levels of 1.8 mg/liter.
Glutethimide	Same	10-80: usually greater than 30 potentially toxic	Nausea; pancytopenia; thrombocytopenia; peripheral neuritis; toxic psychosis; laryngospasm; double vision; pupillary dilation; convulsions; coma
Gold Salts (Aurothioglucose)	Same	Incidence of toxic reactions seems variably related to serum levels.	Skin rash; pruritus; skin eruptions; nausea; vomiting; proteinuria; hepatitis; dermatitis; photosensitivity (X-ray, U.V. & sunlight); aplastic anemia; chrysiasis
Haloperidol	Same	Variable; range of 0.05-0.5 reported	Extra pyramidal reactions; depression; headache; confusion; vertigo; seizures; hypotension; endocrine malfunction; skin rash
Imipramine	Imipramine and desimpramine	1.0-2.0 and greater	QRS duration 100m sec; unconsciousness; abnormal deep tensor reflexes; respiratory depression; seizures; cardiac arrhythmia; cardiac arrest; coma
Indomethacin	Same	Not fully established, probably in excess of 5.0	Nausea; vomiting; diarrhea; epigastric distress; headache; vertigo; possible toxic hepatitis; high incidence of side effects in persons on therapeutic doses
Lidocaine	Same	6 & greater	Methemoglobinemia; fall in blood pressure; convulsions; atrioventricular block; respiratory failure. CNS adverse effects occur more frequently at levels of 9.0 mg/liter and greater
Lithium	Same	1.5mEq/liter and greater	Diarrhea; vomiting; drowsiness; skin eruptions; muscular weakness; athetotic movements; convulsions; coma; fall in blood pressure; thyroid enlargement; bone marrow depression. Incidence of toxic symptoms increases dramatically with levels in excess of 2.0m Eq/liter
Meperidine	Parent compound plus normeperidine	5	Dyspnea; abrupt and marked fall of blood pressure; soft and rapid pulse; hallucinations; muscle twitching; convulsions
Mephenytoin	5-ethyl-5-phenylhydantoin	20	Hemolytic anemia; aplastic anemia; visual disturbances; fever

TABLE 7. (cont'd)

| Drug | Drug/Metabolite Measured | Toxicological Data | |
		Serum Level, mg/liter	Clinical Findings
Meprobamate	Same	50-200	Hypersensitivity reactions; urticaria; erythematous maculopapular skin rash; fever; peripheral edema; non-thrombocytopenic purpura; convulsions on withdrawal of drug
Methadone	Same	Up to 2; greater than 2 may be fatal	Comatose, with slow, shallow, irregular respiration; pupils may be constricted; blood pressure may be slightly decreased; shock. Nausea and constipation are common at therapeutic doses
Methaqualone	Same	6-30	Nausea; vomiting; dry mouth; transient paresthesia; motor excitation followed by deep coma; rapid variations in pupillary width and reaction to light; hyper-reflexia, muscle fasliculations; tonicclonic convulsions
			Major toxic characteristic is the *nachschlaf*—sleep from which patient can be roused and which persists for 24 or more hours after cessation of other toxic symptoms, due to accumulation of active metabolites
Methotrexate	Same	Dependent upon dosage administered	High potential toxicity, usually dose-related depression of bone marrow; anemia; leukopenia; thrombocytopenia; hepatoxicity; diarrhea and ulcerated stomatitis; hemorrhagic enteritis. High Doses (50 mg/kg or >): Normal Leucovorin Rescue: less than 5 x 10⁻⁷M (48 hr.) Inadequate Leucovorin Rescue: > 5 x 10⁻⁷M (48 hr.) Low Doses (< 50 mg/kg): Therapeutic < 2 x 10⁻⁷M, 1-2 weeks after last dose
Methsuximide	Normethsuximide	40-80	Periorbital edema; proteinuria; hepatic dysfunction; bone marrow aplasia; coma
Nortriptyline	Same	Not fully established; probably 0.50 & greater	QRS duration — 100m sec; unconsciousness; seizures; cardiac arrhythmia; hypotension;cardiac arrest
Oxazepam	Same	Not well established; probably in excess of 2.0	Drowsiness; rash; syncope; ataxia; hypotension

TABLE 7. (cont'd)

Paramethadione	5-ethyl-5-methyl-2,4-oxazolidine-dione	700-1500	Hematuria; neutropenia; agranulocytosis; lupus; myasthenia; blurred vision
Pentobarbital	Same		Clinical Stages
		2-4	(1) Awake, competent; mildly sedated
		6-12	(2) Sedated; reflexes present; prefers sleep; does not cerebrate
		15-20	(3) Comatose, refexes present
		20-30	(4) Comatose areflexive
		30	(5) Comatose; circulatory and/or respiratory difficulty
			These clinical stages do not have definite limits but blend into each other as the patient progresses from stage to stage; the concentration given represents the average range for nontolerant patients.
			The deep tendon reflexes were used as the criteria for presence or absence of reflexes; gag and cough reflexes return at approximately the same time as the deep tendon reflexes.
Phenacemide	Same		Headache; insomnia; rash (scarlatinform); nausea; vomiting; abdominal pain; anorexia; hepatitis; leukopenia; pancytopenia; transient albuminurea
Phenobarbital	Same	50-80	Sleepiness; mental confusion; unsteadiness; coma; shallow respiration; hypotension; cyanosis; pulmonary edema; absent reflexes
Phensuximide	Same	80-150	Nausea; vomiting; muscular weakness; hematuria; neuphrosis
Phenytoin	Same	20-100	Swelling of gums; fever; liver damage; agranulocytosis; lupus syndrome; epidermal necrolysis; cardiac irregularities; tremor; convulsions; drug psychosis. The following levels have been associated with specific chemical findings: Nystagmus: 20-30 mg/liter Ataxia: 30-40 mg/liter Speech disturbance: > 40 mg/liter
Primidone	Same	40-80	Fatigue; drowsiness; vomiting; painful gums. Since active metabolite is phenobarbital, toxic symptoms of phenobarbital may also occur

TABLE 7. (cont'd)

| | | **Toxicological Data** | |
| | | Serum Level, | |
Drug	**Drug/Metabolite Measured**	**mg/liter**	**Clinical Findings**
Procainamide	Same	8 and greater	Irregular pulse; fall of blood pressure; fever; chills; pruritus; malaise; systemic lupus erythematosus; agranulocytosis
Prochlorperazine	Same	1.0-2.0 and greater	Primarily involvement of the extrapyramidal mechanism producing dystonic reactions as spasm of neck muscles, extensor rigidity of back muscles, carpopedal spasm, trismus, and protrusion of the tongue; CNS depression; somnolence; coma; convulsions; fever; hyptotension; dry mouth; ileus
Propoxyphene	Parent Compound and norpropoxyphene	5-20	Course of toxic effects is rapid, leading to convulsions, respiratory depression and coma. Deaths are common with overdoses.
Propranolol	Same	Not fully established	Cardiac failure; hypoglycemia; nausea; diarrhea; dizziness; insomnia; fatigue; alopecia; constipation
Protriptyline	Same	Not fully established	Tachycardia and postural hypotension; dry mouth; dilated pupils; dystonia; ataxia, tremor; vertigo; insomnia; tingling of extremities; skin reactions
Quinidine	Same	>8	Fall of blood pressure; nausea; tinnitus; headache; nystagmus; respiratory failure; urticaria; anaphylactoid reactions; atrioventricular (A-V) block; prolongation of OT interval
Sodium Nitroferricyanide	Thiocyanate	Greater than 50	Tinnitus; blurred vision; delirium; hypotension; metabolic acidosis; dyspnea; headache; vomiting; dizziness; ataxia; loss of consciousness. Coma, pink color, very shallow breathing; poisoning — signs similar to cyanide poisoning. Fatalities have been reported at levels in excess of 200 mg/liter

TABLE 7. (cont'd)

Drug	Active form	Level	Toxic symptoms
Theophylline	Same	Less than 15 15-20 20-25 25-30 30-40 40-50 Greater than 50	Relatively few toxic symptoms observed Nausea; vomiting Nausea; vomiting; diarrhea Nausea; vomiting; diarrhea; tremors; excessive bronchorrhea Seizures Seizures; tachycardia; palpitations Convulsions; death
Thioridazine	Parent compound and mesoridazine	1.0-2.0 and greater	Drowsiness; mild hypotension; hypothermia; tachycardia; nausea; ataxia; anorexia; coma; agranulocytosis; jaundice; skin pigmentation
Tolbutamide	Same	100	Hypoglycemia; nausea; vomiting; weakness; skin eruptions; hyperlipemia; ulcer
Tolmetin	Same	60 and greater	Prolongs bleeding time; retention of water and sodium; mild peripheral edema; gastrointestinal effects including epigastric pain, nausea, vomiting, indigestion, heartburn, constipation, dyspepsia; rash
Triflupromazine	Same	Not established	(Similar to Prochlorperazine)
Trimethadione	Dimethadione	1000	Hematuria; neutropenia; agranulocytosis; lupus; myasthenia; blurred vision; anorexia; nausea; vomiting. May elevate or lower plasma levels of other anticonvulsants given in combination
Valproic acid (Valproate sodium)	Same	Not fully established	
Warfarin	Same (plus some hydroxy-metabolites)	10 and greater	Side effects usually minor — mild diarrhea; major toxicity is hemorrhage, hematuria, gastrointestinal, renal, intracranial, retroperitoneal and other sites

In other words, toxic symptoms may occur while plasma or serum levels appear to be in the therapeutic range. An extension of this table, Table 7 (Correlation of Toxic Effects with Serum and Drug Levels), Expands the information provided in Table 6, and presents data compiled from various compendia as well as personal observations of actual serum levels that may be expected to evoke toxic symptoms. Note that in some cases accurate blood level data is not currently available for correlation with specific toxicological findings.

To serve as an example of a fatal consequence of not understanding the necessities of therapeutic drug monitoring and the need to fully investigate the complex parameters involved in interpreting such levels, the report by Vincent (1978) should prove useful. Briefly, a 70 year old man with known chronic obstructive pulmonary disease was admitted to the hospital because of fever and increasing shortness of breath. Upon examination he was found to be cachectic and tachypneic, with a respiratory rate of 35/min., pulse rate of 112/min., and blood pressure of 110/70 mm Hg. Because the patient was believed to be in acute respiratory failure, therapy was started with assisted ventilation and administration of aminophylline (250 mg intraveniously every six hours) and prednisone (20 mg daily). He did resonably well on this regimen, and by day ten assisted ventilation was no longer needed.

For the next ten days he was maintained on 250 mg of aminophylline intravenously every six hours. His condition improved clinically and he had only mild shortness of breath at rest and a trace of peripheral edema. On the morning of day 17 he was found in an unresponsive state, from which he recovered in a few hours. Various studies offered no clues, and the medication regimen was changed to the administration of 200 mg of theophylline, orally, every six hours during the day, and theophylline anhydrous (Slo-Phlline) 250 mg orally at bedtime. Three days later the patient had tonicoclonic epileptic seizure, with associated incontinence and postictal stupor. The seizure began in the left upper extremity, progressed to the right side, and lasted about ten minutes. The results of routine metabolic studies were again noncontributory and a brain scan was normal. Theophylline therapy was discontinued, and a blood sample was sent to the laboratory for a serum theophylline determination. Following a second seizure a short time later, the patient was given 800 mg of phenytoin by slow intravenous infusion, 50 mg/min. He had four more seizures during the afternoon and evening and then lapsed into a stupor. The attacks continued intermittently throughout the night, and the next morning he had a fatal cardiopulmonary arrest.

The laboratory report, which was not available until three days after the patient's death, showed a serum theophylline level of 32.6 mg/liter (normal therapeutic level 10 to 20 mg/liter).

The conclusion reached in the report was that serum theophylline levels should be monitored in patients undergoing medical treatment, particularly when hepatic or circulatory dysfunction co-exists.

3. What Drug Levels Should Be Measured

DRUGS AND THEIR METABOLITES

The metabolism of drugs usually takes place in two distinct phases: Phase I included reactions such as oxidation, reduction, hydrolysis, and various metabolic transformations, and Phase II the conjugation of various metabolites. In Phase I, groups such as OH, COOH, and NH_2 are introduced into the drug molecule. In Phase II, the Phase I metabolite reacts with an endogenous substrate, such as amino acids or glucuronic acids, to yield what is referred to as a conjugated metabolite which is usually excreted from the body. Drugs are usually lipid-soluble compounds and are therefore able to penetrate cell membranes, which are lipoprotein barriers. In general, the more lipid-soluble the drug, the greater is the proportion reabsorbed in the kidney into the tubule cells. The driving force is the concentration gradient produced during reabsorption of water and solutes. The majority of the drug biotransformation reactions are carried out *in vivo* by enzymes which are located in the smooth endoplasmic reticulum of the hepatic cells. The result of metabolic transformation of drugs is metabolites that are more polar and less lipid soluble (therefore more water soluble and easily excreted) than the parent drug.

Although a detailed discussion of the various pathways are beyond the scope of this text, Table 8 lists an overall review of the various metabolic reactions for selected drugs and the transformations taking place. The reader is referred to references such as Drayer (1974), LaDu et al. (1971), Goldstein et al., (1974) and Blaschke (1977) for more detailed information on the metabolic processes various drug compounds.

If a drug has an active metabolite(s), determination of the parent drug alone may cause misleading interpretations of blood level measurement. The plasma level of the pharmacologically active metabolite should also be measured as its biologic half life taking it into account in any decision based upon the determination of drug level assay. Those metabolities with significant pharmocologic activity and demonstrating high plasma levels will probably contribute substantially to the pharmacologic effect ascribed to the parent drug. Table 9 presents a selective listing of drugs that are known to possess pharmocologic active metabolite(s). Table 10 demonstrates how the specific process of demethylation of many of the anti-convulsive drugs in common use today form active metabolites. For example, the measurement of trimethadione without the active metabolite, dimethadione, will provide little useful data. In practice, the measurement of both the parent compound and the active metabolite must be undertaken and the ratio of metabolite to parent compound of 7 to 1 (or greater) achieved until pharmacologic efficacy can be assumed to be effective. Thus, the measurement of mephenytoin, for example, would again

TABLE 8. Selected Examples of Metabolic Reactions of Drugs[1]

I. Synthetic

A. CONJUGATION

1. **With acetic acid:**
   sulphanilamide→N_4-acetylsulphanilamide
   INH→acetyl - INH
   p-aminosalicylic acid→p-acetamidosalicylic acid

2. **With glucuronic acid:**
   phenol→phenolglucuronide
   salicylic acid→0-carboxyphenyl glucuronide
   meprobamate→meprobamate glucuronide

3. **With glycine:**
   benzoic acid→hippuric acid
   nicotinic acid→nicotinuric acid

4. **With sulphate ions:**
   phenol→phenolsulphate
   estrone→estrone sulfate

B. METHYLATION

1. **N-methylation:**
   noradrenaline→adrenaline
   nicotinic acid→N-methylnicotinic acid

2. **O-methylation:**
   adrenaline→methyladrenaline

II. Degradative

C. HYDROLYSIS

1. **Ester cleavage:**
   procaine→aminobenzoic acid + diethylaminoethanol
   meperidine→meperidinic acid + ethanol
   cocaine→benzoylecgonine + CH_3OH

2. **Cleavage of acids from amides:**
   phenacetin→phenetidin + acetic acid
   procainamide→aminocenzoic acid + diethylaminoethylamine

---

[1]Modified from Lembeck (1969).

TABLE 8. (cont'd)

3. **Hydralytic ring cleavage:**

   hesperidin→3-hydroxy-4-methoxy-phenylpropionic acid

D. OXIDATION

1. **C-hydroxylation:**

   meprobamate→hydroxymeprobamate
   barbital→5-ethyl-5-β-hydroxyethylbarbituric acid
   chloral hydrate→trichloroacetic acid
   hexobarbital→ketohexobarbital

2. **Oxidative deamination:**

   amphetamine→phenylacetone + ammonia (benzyl methyl ketone)
   histamine→imidazole acetic acid

3. **Oxidative dealkylation:**

   phenacetin→paracetamol + CH_3CHO
   codeine→morphine

4. **N-Oxidation:**

   aniline→phenylhydroxylamine
   imipramine→imipramine N-oxide

5. **S-Oxidation:**

   chlorpromazine→chlorpromazine sulphoxide
   thioridazine→thioridazine sulfoxide
   thioridazine sulfoxide→thioridazine disulfoxide
   thioridazine disulfoxide→thioridazine sulfone

6. **Oxidative dehalogenation:**

   halothane→trifluoroacetic acid
   methoxyflurane→1,1-difluoroethyl methyl ether

7. **Hydroxylation of aromatic rings:**

   phenylbutazone→oxyphenbutazone
   salicylic acid→gentisic acid
   chlorpromazine→7-hydroxychlorpromazine

8. **N-Dealkylation:**

   imipramine→desmethylimipramine
   meperidine→normeperidine
   mephobarbital→phenobarbital + HCHO

9. **Desulfuration:**

   thiopental→pentobarbital

TABLE 9. Drugs with Pharmacologically Active Metabolites[1]

Parent Drug	Active Metabolite
Acetohexamide	Hydroxyhexamide
Allopurinol	Alloxanthine
Amitriptyline	Nortriptyline
Carbamazepine	Carbamazepine-10,11 Epoxide
Chloral Hydrate	Trichloroethanol
Chlordiazepoxide	Desmethylchlordiazepoxide
	Demoxepam
Clonazepam	7-Aminoclonazepam
Clorazepate	Nordiazepam
Codeine	Morphine
Diazepam	Desmethyldiazepam
Digitoxin	Digoxin
Doxepin	Desmethyldoxepin
Flurazepam	Desalkylflurazepam
Glutethimide	4-hydroxyglutethimide
Imipramine	Desipramine
Lidocaine	Monoethylglycinexylidide
Meperidine	Normeperidine
Mephenytoin	5-ethyl-5-phenylhydantoin
Mephobarbital	Phenobarbital
Metharbital	Barbital
Methamphetamine	Amphetamine
Methsuximide	N-Desmethylmethsuximide
Nitroprusside	Thiocyanate
Paramethadione	5-ethyl-5-methyl-2,4-oxazolidine-dione
Phenacetin	Acetaminophen
Phensuximide	N-Desmethylphensuximide
Phenylbutazone	Oxyphenbutazone
Prednisone	Prednisolone
Primidone	Phenobarbital
	Phenylethylmalonamide
Procainamide	N-acetylprocainamide
Propanolol	4-hydroxypropranolol
Spironolactone	Canrenone
	Canrenoate
Sulfasalazine	Sulfapyridine
Trimethadione	Dimethadione

[1]Reprinted from Morrell and Pribor (1978) with permission from Laboratory Management, 16(7):15-27, 1978.

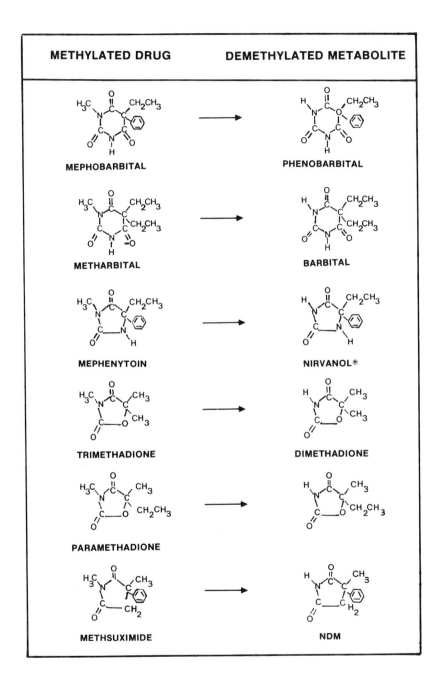

TABLE 10. N-Demethylation of Anticonvulsant Drugs to Form Active Metabolites[1]

[1]From Atkinson and Strong (1977) with grateful permission from the authors and The Plenum Publishing Corp., N.Y.C., N.Y.

provide little useful data, because of the short half-life of the parent compound, and also because essentially all of the parent compound is rapidly metabolized to an active metabolite which in fact accumulates in the plasma and to which has been ascribed the total pharmacologic effect of this particular compound.

Table 11 cites the more commonly used anticonvulsants in man, with their known metabolites that are amenable to assay in drug monitoring. It should be noted that each anti-convulsant has specific uses in the treatment of seizures and epilepsy and both the measurement of parent compound and metabolite may provide the most useful data for seizure control.

The smooth endoplasmic reticulum or microsomal fraction of the liver cells is the major site for the biotransformation (metabolism) of drugs, involving hydroxylation, dealkalinazation, and glucuronic conjugation. Certain drugs can alter this biotransformation by stimulating or otherwise influencing the microsomal enzymes, and can thereby affect the duration and intensity of action of those drugs metabolized by liver microsomes.

TABLE 11. Anticonvulsants and Known Metabolites Measured in Plasma[1]

Drug	Measured Metabolite(s)	Anticonvulsant Action of Metabolite
Ethosuximide	—	—
Methsuximide	N-Desmethylmethsuximide	Yes
Tridione	Dimethadione	Yes
Valproic acid	—	—
Diazepam	Desmethyldiazepam	Yes
	Oxazepam	Negligible at levels produced
Nitrazepam	7-Amino and	
	7-Acetamido-Derivatives	?
Clonazepam	7-Amino-Derivatives	?
Phenobarbital	—	—
Methylphenobarbital	Phenobarbital	Yes
Primidone	Phenylethylmalonamide	Yes
	Phenobarbital	Yes
Carbamazepine	10, 11-Epoxycarbamazepine	Yes
Phenytoin	5-p-Hydroxyphenytoin	No

[1]Adapted from Eadie (1976) with grateful permission from Dr. M.J. Eadie and The ADIS Press.
[2]The dash (—) refers to the fact that there are no measured metabolites and presumably no pharmacologic action of metabolites while the question marks (?) refer to the fact that the anticonvulsant action of these metabolites has not been thoroughly established.

Enzyme induction increases the rate of metabolism of many drugs, and a variety of drugs induce an increase in microsomal enzymes. Several hundred compounds, including hypnotics, anti-convulsants, and antihistamines, are known to stimulate metabolism of drugs when administered to humans. Enzyme induction by a drug is often recognized in patients by the exaggerated, depressed, or adverse effect of another drug concurrently administered. For example, phenobarbital, when administered simultaneously with warfarin and bishydroxycoumarin, has lead to a deep increase in the plasma levels and anticoagulant activity of these agents. If an enzyme-inducing hypnotic drug is given to a patient at the same time he is being titrated with warfarin, he may hemorrhage when the hypnotic drug is discontinued, unless the dose of the anticoagulant is reduced (see Table 36, page 163, for additional examples).

Drug Distribution

A common approach to studying the pharmacokinetic behavior of drugs in the biological system is to depict the body as a system of compartments. In many instances these compartments have no physiologic meaning but are useful in describing the time course of drug levels in the plasma after administration of the drug. Three frequently used compartmental models are normally used. The one compartment model assumes that a drug entering the body is distributed instantaneously into the available space. The one compartment model is particularly useful for describing the time course that most drugs follow in the plasma or urine after oral or intramuscular administration. However, it may or may not adequately describe the time course of the drug in the body after intravenous administration. The adequacy of the model depends on the frequency of plasma sampling after injection of the drug. With frequent plasma samples it is apparent that a more complex model is needed to describe the pharmacokinetics of most drugs.

In most cases, the two compartment open model has been sufficient to describe the pharmacokinetics of these drugs. The model assumes that a drug entering the body instantaneously and homogenously distributes into a space termed the central compartment which consists of the blood and other readily accessible tissues and fluids. Distribution into the rest of the available body space, or peripheral compartment, is somewhat slower. The term "central compartment" can be frequently applied to such physiological areas as the extracellular space and the well perfused organs such as kidney and liver. The peripheral, or tissue compartment, may be considered to consist of poorly perfused organs and tissues such as muscle or fat. In addition, the assumption is often made that drug elimination occurs in the central compartment. A somewhat more complex model consists of a central compartment, connected to two peripheral compartments, which differ in their relative accessibility to a drug.

In describing the processes associated with each model, it is often assumed that they follow first order kinetics, where the rate of a given process is proportional to the amount or concentration of the drug. In the one compartment model the plasma concentration is directly proportional to the amount of drug in the body. A relationship similar to the one compartment model also describes the blood level versus time curve in the two compartment model, once apparent distribution equilibrium between the central and peripheral compartment has been established.

Of prime importance in determining the duration of drug action in the body is the biologic half-life $(t_1/_2)$ of the drug. The data obtained from the careful planning and measurement of the plasma levels, urinary excretion studies, and pharmacologic effect can be used to gain estimates of the biological half-life, that is, the time required to reduce a given plasma concentration to 50% of that level. A further discussion of the utility and the usefulness of the biologic half-life will be undertaken in Chapter 4.

Another useful pharmacokinetic parameter is the apparent volume of distibution of the drug. The apparent volume of distribution of the drug is defined as the amount of drug in the body dividied by the concentration of the drug in the blood. The assumption is made that the body acts as a single homogenuous compartment with respect to the drug. The apparent volume of distribution acts as a proportionality constant between the amount of drug in the body and the concentration of drug in the blood or plasma. Therefore, the volume of distribution (V_d) merely represents a volume calculated by sampling of a reference compartment for the drug. Often, the value of V_d is characteristic of a drug and is constant over a wide dose range. However, this constant may vary under special and unusual circumstances. For example, with drugs that are highly protein bound (to be discussed in the next paragraph), the V_d may be greater at higher doses, as sites of drugs binding to the protein become saturated (see equation 20, page 154, for calculation).

Body fluids in man is comprised of intracellular and extracellular fluid, the extracellular being further subdivided into serum and interstitial fluid. Since drug concentration in the extracellular fluid is in equilibrium with the drug concentration in serum water, the drug concentration in this serum, i.e., free drug concentration, is an indirect measure of the drug concentration at the site of pharmacologic action. In theory, for example, since anticonvulsant drug compounds present in extracellular fluid can cross tissue membranes and ellicit these pharmacologic effects on specific sites of action, the measurement of drug concentration in serum water should be a closer measure of the drug concentration at the site of action than drug concentration in serum. However, in routine practice, serum water drug concentrations have until recently been rarely measured, due primarily to the expense of the additional separation procedures and instrumental sensitivity required for such measurements. Consequently, the measurement of serum drug concentrations is used to reflect the equilibrium between intercellular fluids, extracellular fluids, and serum water concentrations, with the pharmacologic effect for most drugs tending to be proportional to the total serum level of drug.

Protein Binding

The rate of exchange of drugs from one anatomical or morphological fluid compartment to another depends upon many factors such as pK_a of the drug, pH of the fluid compartment, and the extent of protein binding of the particular drug. Since as noted above, the free drug concentration in serum water is a fairly constant percentage of the total drug concentration in serum, the analysis of and pharmacological response remains fairly reliable in these circumstances. However, a high degree of drug binding to various proteins in serum changes the implication of many pharmacokinetic parameters. Drugs may complex with nuclear proteins and interfere with protein synthesis, they may bind with a receptor protein and elicit a pharmacologic response, they may interact with enzymes altering such enzyme activity, or they may complex with plasma or tissue proteins. The binding of a drug to plasma and tissue proteins can influence the distribution of the drug, the rate at which it passes to the membranes, and the intensity of its pharmacologic effect and its elimination rate. An important consideration is the influence that a second drug may have on the protein binding of the first. Drugs with a high association constant or a high affinity for protein may compete for binding sites occupied by other drugs. For example, if two drugs compete for the same binding site, the one with less affinity will be displaced, resulting in a higher concentration of free drug. Only the free (not protein bound drug) is available for drug site or receptor interaction and is pharmacologically active. The increased amount of free drug may result in toxicity, for example, displacement of warfarin by phenybutazone resulting in a hemorrhagic condition. Another example of the consequences of protein binding of various drugs is that the higher the protein binding of a drug, the more severe a toxic reaction is expected upon displacement of when the protein concentration is reduced. Thus, a total serum phenytoin concentration in the normal therapeutic range could be toxic in a patient with renal failure, because he would have an abnormally high serum (and tissue) concentration of free active phenytoin. Whenever the degree of binding of a drug in serum is abnormal or changing, analysis of its pharmacokinetic fate becomes quite complex.

Table 12 presents a representative listing of frequently monitored therapeutic agents which show a high affinity for protein binding, and thus a strong tendency to displace other drugs from protein-bound sites.

Protein binding is also the reason that certain drugs require higher loading doses and why lower maintenance doses have to be given. The practical consequences of active protein binding and other factors is that the dose sizes of repeated dosage should be equal to the amount of the compound which can be adequately metabolized by the body or eliminated from the body. It must be remembered that only the free drug, unbound by any proteins can exert a pharmacological reaction by interaction with the specific site of action. Thus it is important that in any of these instances where changing of the protein binding or possible drug interaction occurs that closely monitored serum samples be taken to reflect the total amount of the drug presently in serum.

Table 12. Selected Drugs that Displace Certain Other Drugs from Protein-Binding Sites in the Serum

Acetaminophen	Nalidixic acid
p-Aminobenzoic acid	Oxyphenbutazone
Barbiturates	Phenylbutazone
Chloral Hydrate	Phenytoin
Clofibrate	Salicylates
Cyclophosphamide	Sulfinpyrazone
Diazoxide	Sulfonamides
Ethacrynic acid	Tolbutamide
Indomethacin	Triiodothyronine
Mefenamic acid	Valproic acid

A practical example of interaction of two drugs competing for a protein binding site is the example of digoxin-quinidine interaction. Various studies have reported that plasma concentrations of digoxin increase approximately two-fold when quinidine is administered along with digoxin. Dr. Hager and his co-workers (Hager et al., 1979) demonstrated that the displacement of digoxin from the binding site occurred in tissue by the action of quinidine causing a rise in the plasma concentration of digoxin. Digoxin toxicity appears to be enhanced in the presence of quinidine, therefore decreasing digoxin dosage is suggested when the drugs are given concurrently. Frequent assessment of the plasma concentration of digoxin and careful attention to the clinical symptoms of toxicity are to be suggested when the two drugs are given in combination.

Table 13 relates the degree of protein (albumin) binding of selected therapeutically monitored drugs.

TABLE 13. Serum Protein Binding of Selected Drugs

Drug	Protein Binding (%)
Acetaminophen	20-50
Amikacin	30
Amobarbital	34
Amphetamine	—
Amitriptyline	80-95
Aprobarbital	50-75
Carbamazepine	60-73
Carbamazepine-10, 11-expoxide	—
Chlordiazepoxide	—
Chlorpromazine	80
Chonazepam	82
Desipramine	High (variable)
Diazepam	96

TABLE 13 (cont.)

Drug	Protein Binding (%)
Desmethyldiazepam	—
Digitoxin	97
Digoxin	23
Dimethadione	—
Disopyramide	—
Doxepin	—
Ethosuximide	0
Ethotoin	—
Flurazepam	—
N-Desalkyl-flurazepam	—
Gentamicin	30
Glutethimide	50
Haloperidol	70
Imipramine	High (variable)
Indomethacin	90
Isoniazid	15
Lidocaine	66
Monoethylglycine-xylidide	60
Lithium	0
Meperidine	40
Mephenytoin	20-50
Mephobarbital	—
Methadone	87
Methotrexate	50
Methsuximide	0
Normethsuximede	0
Nortriptyline	High (variable)
Paramethadione	0
5-ethyl-5methyl-2, 4-oxazolidine-dione	0
Pentobarbital	35-45
Phenobarbital	45-50
Phesuximide	—
Phenytoin	88
Primidone	0-30
Phenylethyl-malonamide	—
Procainamide	15
N-acetyl-procainamide	—
Propranolol	93
4-hydroxy-propranolol	—
Quinidine Gluconate	—
Quinidine Sulfate	82
Salicylic acid	50-90
Sulfadiazine	45
Sulfamethoxazole	68
Sulfisoxazole	86
Theophylline	15
Tobramycin	10
Tolbutamide	50-80
Trimethadione	0
Dimethadione	0
Valproic acid	90-100
Warfarin	97

58

4. When Should Serum Levels Be Monitored?

Timing of Measurements

The biologic half-life ($t_{1/2}$ of the drug) is of prime importance when determining the duration of the drug action in the body. The half-life and elimination rate constant are dependent upon two important factors: the volume of distribution (V_d) and the total clearance of the drug from the body. It is clear that the $t_{1/2}$ may be shortened by reduction in the volume of distribution, by enhanced clearance, or by a combination of these changes. Conversely, $t_{1/2}$ may be prolonged when the value of distribution is increased, the clearance diminished, or both. The $t_{1/2}$ may remain the same when changes in clearance in the volume of distribution exactly balance each other. The half-life therefore depends on both the amount of plasma or tissue cleared of a drug in a given time and the distribution of the drug throughout the tissues. Of practical importance are those patients which have increased or decreased clearances, hence prolonging or decreasing the $t_{1/2}$, thus increasing or decreasing the actual plasma levels of the pharmacologic active drugs.

The dosage interval depends on the half-life of the drug, the safety or therapeutic index of the drug, the character of the concentration-response curve, and the minimum effective plasma concentration. A note of caution— when dealing with multicompartmental models, it is important to note that the biologic half-life is a functional value obtained in the distribution equilibrium phase and that this phase does not represent the true elimination rate but rather a hybrid constant consisting of the parameters of distribution and elimination.

The half-life of a drug is an extremely useful parameter to use to adjust the dosage regime of a therapeutic agent. Drugs with large $t_{1/2}$ may be administered with less frequency (as with many of the anticonvulsants or antidepressants), than drugs with relatively short half lives. For example, the dosing of phenytoin with its 20 hour half-life and nortriptyline with its 20 to 60 hour half-life may be done on once a day basis. A practical outcome of this type of dosage may be greater patient compliance as the frequency of dose is decreased. As a general rule, the best time to take a drug sample for therapeutic monitoring is just before the next dose ("trough" level). This would apply to drugs given on a regular schedule.

The patient should have been subjected to a regimen of drug therapy for a long enough period of time to be in a steady state as regards drug intake and elimination before drug levels in serum are measured. For drugs which are eliminated according to processes which follow mono-exponential kinetics (many of the anticonvulsants and antidepressants), vitually steady state plasma levels are achieved within 5 'drug half lives'(see Biological half-life in Glossary. Thus, this period should elapse before plasma antidepressant or anticonvulsant levels are measured. However, when, for example, an anticonvulsant dose is held constant, but the dose of another drug is changed, it is difficult to provide any general rule as to when plasma anticonvulsant levels will again become steady, should the other drug alter the body's distribution, metabolism, or excretion of the anticonvulsant. Diminished activity of hepatic drug-metabolizing enzymes, for example, might occur over some weeks after a drug is stopped, and the clinician must bear this possibility in mind when ordering and interpreting plasma anticonvulsant (and other drugs) measurements after change in dosage of another drug.

Most drugs with extended half lives should be sampled once the patient has reached a plateau or steady state level arrived at in about five times the half-life. There are special circumstances when both the peak levels and trough levels of a drug should be obtained. For example, patients receiving aminoglycosides (tobramycin, gentamycin, amakicin) should have both a peak and a trough serum level measured after 3 to 5 doses and again on the fifth day of therapy (Jackson, 1977; Noone, 1978; Flynn et al., 1978). While not all investigators agree as to whether elevated peak serum levels predict toxicity, it is clear that they indicate whether therapeutic levels have been achieved. Increasing trough levels may indicate accumulation of the drug due to impaired renal function and thus call for an alteration of dosage. In the case of aminoglycoside therapy, serum levels should be performed twice a week in patients with normal renal failure and more frequently in those with renal insufficiency. Peak and trough level determinations should be made 24 hours after any change in aminoglycoside dosage to insure therapeutic levels.

Dr. Sanders (1980) has cited these indications for monitoring serum concentrations of aminoglycosides:

1. Patients with normal renal failure to assure that peak levels are in the therapeutic range and that trough levels are not excessive.

2. Patients with impaired renal function and/or rapidly changing renal function.

3. Patients undergoing dialysis.

4. Patients who are not responding to therapy.

5. Patients who have not received more than five days' treatment—even those without obvious impaired renal function.

6. Patients who develop symptoms and/or signs of ototoxicity or nephrotoxicity.

7. Patients with aerobic gram-negative bacteria or gram-negative pneumonia or both.

8. Patients with burns or cystic fibrosis.

9. Patients who are elderly because creatinine clearance provides only a rough estimation of glomerular function, which tends to decrease with age.

10. Patients with conditions associated with lower peak level—fever, obesity, and expanded extracellular fluid volume.

As another example, digoxin represents a special circumstance where distribution from blood into tissues takes 6 to 8 hours and a blood sample for digoxin should not be taken during this period. Also, many other drugs may be given in low dose. Typically, for example, digoxin may be given in amounts up to 1 mg or more on the first day of treatment. In such case, the blood level would be more informative if taken six hours or more after the last loading dose as opposed to calculating sampling time on the basis of biological half- life. Serum levels should be measured in a steady state time and fixed times in relation to the drug dosage interval. Table 14 sets forth data on biologic half-life of selected drugs and their metabolites. Table 15 expands the data of Table 14 with some selected exceptions to provide the physician with the actual recommended time of sampling and whether this is the peak or trough levels.

TABLE 14. Biological Half-Lives of Selected Drugs and Metabolites

Drug	Biological Half-Life ($t_{1/2}$), Hrs.	References
Acetaminophen	1-4	Albert, K.S., et al. (1974a) Albert, K.S., et al. (1974b) Levy, G., and Yamada, H. (1971)
Amikacin	2-3	Clarke, J.T. et al. (1974)
Amobarbital	13-45	Kadar, D. et al. (1973) Clifford, J.M. et al. (1974)
Amphetamine	7-140 (urine ph>6.6) 18-34.0 (urine ph <6.6)	Anggard, E. et al. (1973) Hinsvark, O.N. et al. (1973) Davis, J.M. et al. (1971) Anggard, E. et al. (1970) Rowland, M. (1969) Wilkinson, G.R. and Beckett, A.H. (1968a) Wilkinson, G.R. and Beckett, A.H. (1968b) Kuntzman, R.G. et al. (1971)
Amitriptyline	15-25	Asberg, M. et al. (1971)
Aprobarbital	0.5-1.5 days	Lous, P. (1954a)
Barbital	2.4-3.3 days	Lous, P. (1954a) Lous, P. (1954b)
Carbamazepine	10-28	Pippenger, C.E. et al. (1978) Palmer, L. et al. (1973)
Carbamazepine-10, 11-epoxide	5-16	Pippenger, C.E. et al. (1978) Palmer, L. et al. (1973)
Chlordiazepoxide	5-20	Schwartz, M.A. et al. (1971)
Chlorpromazine	16-30	Maxwell, J.D. et al. (1972)
Clonazepam	13-46	Pippenger, C.E. et al. (1978) Dreifuss, F.E. et al. (1975)
Desipramine	12-24	Asberg, M. et al. (1971)

TABLE 14 (cont.)

Drug	Biological Half-Life (t½), Hrs.	References
Diazepam	20-40	Pippenger, C.E. et al. (1978) DeSilva, A.J. et al. (1966) Klotz, U. et al. (1975) Hillestad, L. et al. (1974) Kaplan, S.A. et al. (1973) Berlin, A. et al. (1972) Marcus, F.I. (1975)
Desmethyldiazepam	60-95	Pippenger, C.E. et al. (1978) DeSilva, A.J. et al. (1966)
Digitoxin	5-8 days	Rasmussen, K. et al. (1972)
Digoxin	0.7-2.0 days	Storstein, L. (1974) Koup, J.R. et al. (1975) Kramer, W.G. et al. (1974) Marcus, F.I. (1975)
Dimethadione	240	Pippenger, C.E. et al. (1978)
Disopyramide	4-10	Ranney, R.E. et al. (1978)
Doxepin	>12	O'Brien, J.E. and Hinsvark, O.N. (1976)
Ethosuximide	60	Pippenger, C.E. et al. (1978) Buchanan, R.A. et al. (1978)
Ethotoin	3-6	
Flurazepam	24-48	DeSilva, J.A.F., et al. (1974)
N-Desalkyl-flurazepam	24	De Silva, J.A.F., et al. (1974)
Gentamicin	2-4	Lockwood, W.R. and Bower, J.D. (1973) Regamey, C. et al. (1973) Simon, V.K. et al. (1973)
Glutethimide	5-22	Kadar, D. et al. (1973) Curry, S.H. et al. (1971)
Gold	0.5-8 days	Harth, M. (1974)
Haloperidol	13-36	Cressman, W.A. et al. (1974)
Imipramine	8-16	Alexanderson, B. (1972) Gram, L.F. and Christianson, J. (1975)
Indomethacin	2-8	Champion, G.D. et al. (1972) Duggan, D.E. et al. (1972) Alvan, G. and Orme, M. (1975)
Isoniazid	1.0-2.0, rapid acetylator 3.0-3.8 slow acetylator	Jenne, J.W. (1964) Mattila, M.J. et al. (1969) Acocella, G. et al. (1972) Tiitinen, H. (1969) Levi, A.J. et al. (1968)

TABLE 14 (cont.)

Drug	Biological Half-Life (t½), Hrs.	References
Lidocaine	1-2	Thomson, P.D. *et al.* (1973) Boyes, R.N. *et al.* (1971) Rowland, M. *et al.* (1971) Wagner, J.G. (1967)
Monoethylglycine-xylidide	2-4	Rowland, M. *et al.* (1971)
Lithium	10-24	Groth, U. *et al.* (1974) Amdisen, A. and Sjogren, J. (1968)
Meperidine	1.5-4.0	Burns, J.O. *et al.* (1955)
Mephenytion	not established	Pippenger, C.E. *et al.* (1978)
Mephobarbital	1-3	Pippenger, C.E. *et al.* (1978)
Methadone	15-30	Baselt, R.C. and Casarett, L.J., (1972) Inturrisi, C.E. and Verebely, K., (1972)
Methotrexate	1-1.5	Adamson, R.H. (1971)
Methsuximide	1.2-1.6	Pippenger, C.E. *et al.* (1978)
Normethsuximide	28-36	Pippenger, C.E. *et al.* (1978)
Nortriptyline	18-93	Asberg, M. *et al.* (1971) Vesell. E.S. *et al.* (1971) Alexanderson, B. (1972) Hammer, W. *et al.* (1969) Gram, L.F. (1974)
Paramethadione	24-72	
5-ethyl-5-methyl-2-4-oxazolidine-dione	150-300	
Pentobarbital	40-50	Smith, R.B. *et al.* (1973) Reidenberg, M.M. *et al.* (1976)
Phenobarbital	50-120	Pippenger, C.E. *et al.* (1978) Garrettson, L.K. and Dayton, P.G., (1970) Butler, T.C. *et al.* (1954)
Phensuximide	6-8.5	Glazko, A.J. and Dill, W.A. (1972)

TABLE 14 (cont.)

Drug	Biological Half-Life (t½), Hrs.	References
Phenytoin	18-22 (Varies according to plasma level due to satuation kinetics.)	Pippenger, C.E. et al. (1978) Serrano, E.E. et al. (1973) Lund, L. et al. (1974) Buchanan, R.A. et al. (1972) Arnold, K. and Gerber. N., (1970) Viukari, N.M.A. and Tammisto P. (1969)
Primidone	6-8	Pippenger, C.E. et al. (1978)
Phenylethyl-malonamide	24-48	Pippenger, C.E. et al. (1978) Gallagher, B.B., et al. (1972)
Procainamide	2.0-4.0	Weily, H.S. and Genton, E. (1972) Koch, Weser, J. and Klein, S.W., (1971)
N-acetyl-procainamide	3.0-6.0	Weily, H.S. and Genton, E. (1972)
Propranolol	3.0-6.0	George, C.F. et al. (1972)
4-hydroxy-propranolol	4.0-8.0	George, C.F. et al. (1972) Fitzgerld, J.D. and O'Donnell, S.R. (1971)
Quinidine Gluconate	3.0-16.0	Kessler, K.M. et al. (1974)
Quinidine Sulfate	7.2	Goldberg, W.M. and Chakrabarti, S.G. (1964)
Salicylic acid	0.5-30 (dose dependent)	Levy, G. (1965a) Rowland, M. et al. (1972) Rowland, M. and Riegelman, S. (1968) Levy, G. (1965b) Wan, S.H. et al. (1974)
Sulfadiazine	10-20	Madsen, S.T. and Iversen, P.F. (1964)
Sulfadimethoxine	60-70	Madsen, S.T. and Iversen, P.F. (1964) Devrienndt, A. et al. (1970)
Sulfamethazine	7.0	Madsen, S.T. and Iversen, P.F. (1964) Fischer, E. (1972)
Sulfamethoxazole	8-14	Madsen, S.T. and Iversen, P.F. (1964) Kostenbauder, H.B. et al. (1962)
Sulfisoxazole	6.0	Madsen, S.T. and Iversen, P.F. (1964) Kaplan, S.A. et al. (1972)

TABLE 14 (cont.)

Drug	Biological Half-Life $(t_{1/2})$, Hrs.	References
Theophylline	3-8	Mitenko, P.A. and Ogilvie, R.I. (1974) Mitenko, P.A. and Ogilvie, R.I. (1973a) Mitenko, P.A. and Ogilvie, R.I. (1972) Mitenko, P.A. and Ogilvie, R.I. (1973b)
Tobramycin	3-5	Lockwood, W.R. and Bower, J.D. (1973) Regamey, C. et al. (1973) Simon, V.K. et al. (1973)
Tolbutamide	3.5-8.0	Matin, S.B. et al. (1974) Sotaniemi, E. et al. (1971) Nelson, E. (1964)
Trimethadione	16-20	Pippenger, C.E. et al. (1978)
Valproic acid	7-15	Pippenger, C.E. (1977) Loiseau, P., Brachet, et al. (1975)
Warfarin	29-70 (depending on which enantiomorph (R^+) or (S^-) measured)	Levy, G. et al. (1970) Brekenridge, A. et al. (1974) O'Reilly, S.A. (1974)

Clinical Considerations

Although pharmacokinetic considerations determine when plasma drug levels may be monitored most meaningfully in the context of current available knowledge, there remains the question of when the measurements are most useful clinically. The following summarizes some of the clinical indications for monitoring:

   a) At the outset of therapy, to see if a satisfactory plasma drug level has been obtained.
   b) During course of therapy if illness fails to be controlled, or escapes from control.
   c) If intercurrent illness develops.
   d) If dosage is changed.
   e) When symptoms occur which might be due to drug's effect.
   f) If dosage of any other concomitantly administered drug is changed.
   g) During pregnancy.
   h) To help ensure patient compliance during course of therapy.
   i) If dosage formulation is changed.

TABLE 15. Time Sampling Requirements, Time to Peak and Steady-State Levels, and Peak/Trough Data for Selected Monitored Drugs

Generic Drug	Time to Peak Level (Hour)	Time to Steady State (Hour) Adults	Time to Steady State (Hour) Children	Sampling Time Peak	Sampling Time Trough
Acetaminophen	0.5-1.0	10-20	10-20	(See Case History 9, p. 132 for detailed sampling times)	
Acetylsalicylic acid	1.0-2.0	10-23	10-15	No	Yes
Amikacin	[1]	10-15[1]	NE	Yes[1]	Yes[1]
Amitriptyline	4-8	4-8 days	NE	No	Yes
Carbamazepine	6-18	2-6 days	2-4 days	No	Yes
Chloramphenicol	2-3	7-25	NE	No	Yes
Desipramine	2-8	2.5-11 days	NE	No	Yes
Digoxin	1.5-5.0	7-11 days	2-10 days	No	Yes
Disopyramide	0.5-3.0	25-30	NE	No	Yes
Ethosuximide	1-2	8-12 days	6-10 days	No	Yes
Gentamicin	[2]	10-15[2]	10-15[2]	Yes[2]	Yes[2]
Imipramine	1-2	2-5 days	NE	No	Yes
Lidocaine	15-30 min[3]	5-10[3]	NE[3]	Yes[3]	Yes[3]
Lithium	1-3	2-7 days	NE	No	Yes
Methotrexate	1-2[4]	[5]	[5]	No	Yes[5]
Nortriptyline	4-8	4-19 days	NE	No	Yes
Phenobarbital	6-18	11-25 days	8-15 days	No	Yes
Phenytoin	4-8	4-6 days	2-5 days	No	Yes
Primidone	2-4	16-60[6]	20-30[6]	No	Yes
Procainamide	1-2	11-20	NE	Yes[7]	Yes[7]
Propranolol	1-2	10-30 days	NE	No	Yes
Quinidine	1.5-2.0[8]	20-35	NE	Yes[8]	Yes[8]
Theophylline	2-3[9]	15-40	5-40	No	Yes
Tobramycin	[10]	10-15[10]	NE	Yes[10]	Yes[10]
Valproic Acid	2-8	40-75	30-75	No	Yes

[1]Varies according to clinical status of patient, dose regimen, and pathological factors.

[2]Varies according to clinical status of patient, dose regimen, and pathological factors.

[3]Varies according to clinical status of patient, clinical indication, and dosage. Trough levels should be drawn 3-5 hours after administration of drug.

[4]Intravenous dosages reach peak levels in 0.5-1.0 hours.

[5]Varies depending upon route of administration and high or low dose regiments (See Table 7). In high doses specimen is taken after 48 hours, followed by an intravenous Leucovorin "rescue".

[6]Rate dependent upon metabolic process to Phenobarbital.

[7]Peak levels may provide data to measure risk of toxicity, while to measure the potential prophypactic effectiveness of the dose, trough levels are indicated.

[8]The slow release formulations exhibit peak levels in 4-8 hours. (See indication for peak and trough levels for Procainamide.)

[9]Dependent upon dosage form - slow release formulations exhibit peak levels in 3-6 hours.

[10]Varies according to clinical status of patient, dose regimen, and pathological factors.

NE—Data not fully established.

5. Interpretation of Plasma Drug Levels

Concept of Therapeutic Range

Individual as well as temporal differences exist in the processes that determine the relationship between serum drug levels, concentrations at the site of drug action, and efficacy of action. The *serum concentrations of drugs may not in themsleves be perfect indices of the degree of pharmacologic response.* Knowing the serum concentration of a drug, one cannot predict exactly the degree of therapeutic (or toxic) action for an individual patient. The important point is that a more accurate prediction can be made from the serum level than from the dosage. By determining serum concentrations, one at least eliminates the largest source of individual difference in the dosage-effect relationship of may drugs. For this reason, dosage adjustments can often be guided by knowledge of serum levels.

Measurements of serum levels of drugs become useful guides for dosage adjustments only when the therapeutically effective range of serum concentrations has been defined by careful clinical studies. Paradoxically, recognition of the clinical value of knowing serum concentrations of potent drugs must not lend to their uncritical use; *therapeutic* decisions should never be based solely on the drug concentrations in serum or plasma, but should always be interpreted in the context of all clinical data. These factors that must be considered when reviewing blood level determinations include:

1. Dosage
2. Route of administration
3. Gastro-intestinal absorption
4. Weight of the patient
5. Dosage formulation or form
6. Tissue binding and active and inactive sites
7. Body water content
8. Rate of detoxification
9. Rate of elimination
10. Storage
11. Induction or inhibition of microsomal enzymes
12. Sex
13. Menstrual cycle
14. Diseased state
15. Synergistic or antagonistic action of other drugs
16. Tolerance
17. Time of sampling
18. Method of analysis (including metabolites).
19. Patient compliance
20. Drug interactions

Table 16 sets forth various monitored drugs with plasma concentrations noted in relation to pharmacologic response.

Patient Compliance

The most common cause of a low serum concentration is unreliable intake, i.e., the patients do not take the medication as prescribed. Kutt and his co-workers (1966) investigated 16 patients whose serum concentrations of DPH were too low and found that 12 of them did not remember to take their medication. There have been different suggestions for helping them remember: more frequent visits, check of the serum concentration, informing the patient what it was, supplying them with a "medicine-reminder box," and simplifying the schedule so all the medicine is taken in a single dose at bedtime. Increasing the visits and checking the serum concentrations increased the mean serum concentration from 18 to 28 μg/ml in outpatients, the same mean as in inpatients on the same dose.

In a study at Johns Hopkins University the non-compliance rate showed an astonishing 30-40% when detailed histories could be obtained from patients on theophylline therapy. Certainly this is perhaps the most difficult aspect of drug therapy to control, especially with outpatients. It is the role of the physician to instruct and guide patients as to the benefits of medications, even if they "feel all right." Because of the high percentage of non-compliance, all unusual blood level concentrations should be fully investigated with medication histories and viewed in the context of possible non-compliance as an initial step.

The way to ensure the patients take medication consists of knowing the circumstances associated with poor compliance and recognizing the physician's part in planning and explaining treatment.

Some of the possible sources of compliance failures are:

1. Not adequate medical record-keeping.
2. Inadequate nurse supervision of patients receiving drug.
3. Erroneous estimates of deterioration.
4. Medical schools historically have not adjusted themselves (other than 1 or 2 semesters) to the practical problems of clinical pharmacology for the general physician and staff personnel. However, steps are being taken, as evidenced by recent articles published by the AMA, etc., that formalized education is being reorganized and upgraded. Another factor, to upgrade physicians' understanding, is the establishment of clinical pharmacokinetics consultation services in various hospitals (see Taylor et al., 1979; Wilson and Wilkinson, 1974; Levy, 1978).
5. Failure to follow dosage instructions.
6. Medication side effects.
7. Patient often attends physician alone.
8. Uncooperative relatives.

TABLE 16. Plasma Concentrations of Therapeutic Agents in Relation to Pharmacologic Response.[1]

Drug		Drug/Metabolite Measured	Therapeutic Range, MG/Liter	Pharmacologic Indication
Generic Name	Brand Name			
ACETAMINOPHEN	TYLENOL	SAME	10-20	ANALGESIC
AMIKACIN	AMIKIN	SAME	15-30	ANTIBIOTIC
AMITRIPTYLINE	ELAVIL	SAME	0.1-0.3	ANTIDEPRESSANT
		NORTRIPTYLINE	0.05-0.15	ANTIDEPRESSANT
CARBAMAZEPINE	TEGRETOL	SAME	8-12	ANTICONVULSANT
		CARBAMAZEPINE-10,11 EPOXIDE	0.2-2.0	ANTICONVULSANT
CHLORDIAZEPOXIDE	LIBRIUM	SAME	1-2	TRANQUILIZER
		DESMETHYL-CHLORDIAZ-EPOXIDE	0.2-0.5	TRANQUILIZER
		DEMOXEPAM	0.1-0.7	TRANQUILIZER
CHLORPROMAZINE	THORAZINE	SAME	0.03-0.60	TRANQUILIZER
		CPZ-SULFOXIDE	9-30 NG/ML	ANTICONVULSANT
CLONAZEPAM	CLONOPIN	SAME	5-70 NG/ML	ANOREXIC
CLORAZEPATE	TRANXENE	NORDIAZEPAM	0.05-0.50	ANTIDEPRESSANT
DESIPRAMINE	NORPRAMIN	SAME	NOT ESTABLISHED	TRANQUILIZER
DIAZEPAM	VALIUM	SAME	0.05-0.20	TRANQUILIZER
		DESMETHYLDIAZEPAM	0.3-1.2	TRANQUILIZER
		OXAZEPAM	NOT ESTABLISHED	
DIGOXIN	LANOXIN	SAME	1-2 NG/ML	CARDIOVASCULAR
DIMETHADIONE	DIMETHADIONE	SAME	200-800	ANTICONVULSANT
DISOPYRAMIDE	NORPACE	SAME	2-4	ANTIARRHYTHMIC
DOXEPIN	SINEQUAN	SAME	5-50 NG/ML	ANTIDEPRESSANT
		NORDOXEPIN	5-100 NG/ML	ANTIDEPRESSANT
DYPHYLLINE	NEOTHYLLINE/LUFYLLIN	SAME	10-20	BRONCHODILATOR
ETHOSUXIMIDE	ZARONTIN	SAME	40-100	ANTICONVULSANT
ETHOTOIN	PEGANONE	SAME	6-20	ANTICONVULSANT
FLURAZEPAM	DALMANE	SAME	5-20 NG/ML	TRANQUILIZER
		N-DESALKYL-FLURAZEPAM	40-60 NG/ML	TRANQUILIZER
GENTAMICIN	GARAMYCIN	SAME	4-10	ANTIBIOTIC

TABLE 16 (cont.)

Drug		Drug/Metabolite Measured	Therapeutic Range, MG/Liter	Pharmacologic Indication
Generic Name	**Brand Name**			
GLUTETHIMIDE	DORIDEN	SAME	0.2-0.8	SEDATIVE
GOLD SALTS	SOLGANAL	SAME	UP TO 5.0	ANTIARTHRITIC
HALOPERIDOL	HALDOL	SAME	UP TO 50 NG/ML	TRANQUILIZER
IMIPRAMINE	TOFRANIL	SAME	0.05-2.50	ANTIDEPRESSANT
		DESIPRAMINE	1.5-5.0	ANTIDEPRESSANT
ISONIAZID	INH	SAME	0.1-0.9	ANTITUBERCULAR
LIDOCAINE	XYLOCAINE	SAME	1.2-5.0	ANTIARRHYTHMIC
		MONOETHYLGLYCINE-XYLIDIDE	0.5-1.5	ANTIARRHYTHMIC
LITHIUM	ESKALITH	SAME	0.5-1.2 MEQ/LITER	ANTIDEPRESSANT
MEPHOBARBITAL	MEBARAL	SAME	5-15	ANTICONVULSANT
		PHENOBARBITAL	15-30	ANTICONVULSANT
MEPHENYTOIN	MESANTOIN	5-ETHYL-5-PHENYL-HYDANTOIN	6-20	ANTICONVULSANT
METHSUXIMIDE	CELONTIN	SAME	0.1-1.4	ANTICONVULSANT
		NORMETHSUXIMIDE	10-40	ANTICONVULSANT
NORTRIPTYLINE	AVENTYL	SAME	0.05-0.15	ANTIDEPRESSANT
PARAMETHADIONE	PARADIONE	SAME	UP TO 10	ANTICONVULSANT
		5-ETHYL-5-METHYL-2,4-OXAZOLIDINE-DIONE	75-750	ANTICONVULSANT
PHENOBARBITAL	ESKABARB	SAME	15-40	ANTICONVULSANT
PHENSUXIMIDE	MILONTIN	SAME	30-60	ANTICONVULSANT
PHENYTOIN	DILANTIN	SAME	10-20	ANTICONVULSANT
PRIMIDONE	MYSOLINE	SAME	5-12	ANTICONVULSANT
		PHENOBARBITAL	12-40	ANTICONVULSANT
		PHENYLETHYL-MALONAMIDE	5-12	ANTICONVULSANT
PROCAINAMIDE	PRONESTYL	SAME	4-8	ANTIARRHYTHMIC
		N-ACETYL-PROCAINAMIDE	2-6	ANTIARRHYTHMIC

TABLE 16 (cont.)

| Drug | | | | |
Generic Name	Brand Name	Drug/Metabolite Measured	Therapeutic Range, MG/Liter	Pharmacologic Indication
PROPRANOLOL	INDERAL	SAME	35-250 NG/ML	β-ADRENERGIC BLOCKER
		4-HYDROXY-PROPRANOLOL	8-70 NG/ML	β-ADRENERGIC BLOCKER
QUINIDINE	QUINIDEX	SAME	3-6	ANTIARRHYTHMIC
SALICYLATE	ASPIRIN	SAME	50-100	ANALGESIC
		SAME	150-300	ANTIARTHRITIC
THEOPHYLLINE	ELIXOPHYLLIN	SAME	10-20	BRONCHODILATOR
THIORIDAZINE	MELLARIL	SAME	0.05-0.30	TRANQUILIZER
		MESORIDAZINE	0.20-1.50	TRANQUILIZER
TOBRAMYCIN	NEBCIN	SAME	3-10	ANTIBIOTIC
TOLBUTAMIDE	ORINASE	SAME	50-95	ANTIDIABETIC
TRIMETHADIONE	TRIDIONE	SAME	UP TO 20	ANTICONVULSANT
		DIMETHADIONE	200-800	ANTICONVULSANT
VALPROIC ACID	DEPAKENE	SAME	60-130	ANTICONVULSANT

¹Reprinted from Morrell and Pribor (1978) with permission from Laboratory Management, 16(7):15-27, 1978.

9. Non-compliance, particularly where no untoward or toxic symptoms have developed, may be a factor where familiar surroundings and a strict schedule has been followed. This may be the case in any routine or habitual process maintained over a long time (Anderson et al., 1976; Wilson and Wilkinson, 1974).
10. No previous attacks after withdrawal of medication.
11. Patient has no system for remembering to take medication.
12. Irregular intake of medication.
13. Other negatively motivating environmental data, might include simple forgetfulness, lack of apparent benefit of medication, large numbers of medications being taken at the same time, and many socio-economic factors, including poverty and isolation (Bochner et al., 1978).
14. Habitual behavior patterns of not taking medication.

Combined Drug Action

Drug interaction may fall into three main classifications:

1. **Pharmacokinetic Interaction**: Drugs that may affect the absorption, distribution, metabolism, or excretion of other drugs. An example is plasma protein binding alteration. Table 17 illustrates a selective group of drugs which can inhibit the metabolism of a primary drug thus resulting in its intoxication.

TABLE 17. Selected Drug Intoxications Caused by Inhibition of Drug Metabolism[1]

Active	Inhibitory Agent	Symptoms of Toxicity
Chlorpropamide	Dicumarol	Hypoglycemic collapse
Chlorpropamide	Phenylbutazone	Hypoglycemic collapse
Phenytoin	Dicumarol	Vertigo, anorexia
Phenytoin	Disulfiram	Cerebellar symptoms
Phenytoin	Phenylbutazone	Vertigo, anorexia, vomiting
Phenytoin	Sulthiame	Vertigo, anorexia, vomiting
Tolbutamide	Dicumarol	Hypoglycemic collapse
Tolbutamide	Chloramphenicol	Hypoglycemic collapse
Tolbutamide	Phenylbutazone	Hypoglycemic collapse

[1]Adapted from Kristensen (1976) with permission of the author and The ADIS Press.

2. **Pharmacologic Interactions**: Synergistic and/or antagonistic effects.

Under this category drug interactions may be classified as:

a. INDIFFERENT: The presence of both drugs results in a biological effect representing the action of each drug unaffected by the presence of the other.

b. SYNERGISM: This describes an effect of two drugs whose combined action is greater than that which can be explained by the additive effect of both drugs.

c. ANTAGONISM: The presence of one drug interferes with and reduces the biological activity of another.

The above three interactions of drugs are usually more readily demonstrated *in vitro* with antibiotics. For example, synergistic activity between trimethoprim and sulphafurazole can be demonstrated on an inoculated medium with *P. morganii* (Waterworth, 1978). Scherr and his co-workers (Scherr and Bechtle, 1959; Bechtle and Scherr, 1959) have also reported methods for *in vitro* assessment of the synergistic and antagonistic effect of various chemical agents in enhancing antimicrobial activity. Drug interactions have been well discussed in texts by Hansten, 1975; Hartshorn, 1976; and Martin, 1978.

3. **Other Interactions**: Drug interactions not falling into the above two previous categories, such as food—drug interactions (Hansten, 1955).

The complexity of possible drug-drug interactions can be gleaned from the following example:

An adverse reaction of lithium with hydrochlorothiazide can result in reversible electrocardiographic abnormalities and physical signs and symptoms of lithium toxicity (Haynes and Elmore, 1979). Since lithium is excreted almost exclusively through the kidneys, the serum level of the drug is determined by the particular maintenance dose, as well as the renal elimination of the compound. Hence, concomitant administration of lithium and thiazide, or a thiazide-diuretic which acts on the distal convoluted tubule, may result in an adverse reaction (Jefferson and Kalin, 1979). These diuretics reduce renal lithium clearance, including lithium retention to potentially toxic serum levels causing amorexia, apathy, muscle twitching, atoxia, and dysarthia. Therefore, whenever feasible, the lithium dose may have to be lowered and the levels more closely monitored to eliminate toxicity (Peterson et al., 1974).

As a final example of possible drug interaction, in this case a drug interaction between a particular drug and a constituent of a foodstuff, the example of phenacetin and charcoal-broiled beef may be representative. Patients who took phenacetin after eating charcoal-broiled beef had for several days markedly lower plasma concentrations of phenacetin, although plasma levels of N-acetyl-p-amino-phenol (APAP, the major metabolite of phenacetin) were not significantly altered.

The markedly decreased bio-availability of phenacetin, after a char-coal-broiled beef diet, was not accompanied by an appreciable change in the plasma level for phenacetin or urinary excretion of APAP. These findings indicate that charcoal-broiled beef stimulated the metabolism of phenacetin probably due to the polycyclic aro-matic hydrocarbons which are extremely potent inducers of certain drug metabolizing enzymes in the gastrointestinal tract and/or dur-ing its first passage through the liver (Conney et al., 1976).

Table 18 presents some of the drug-drug interactions that can drastically alter various plasma levels and hence the interpretations of whether toxic or thera-peutic levels are truly being developed.

TABLE 18. Selected Drug-Drug Interactions with Practical Implications for Therapeutic Drug Monitoring of Plasma Drug Levels

Drug Class	Measured Drug	Interacting Drug	Effect	Reference
ANTIDEPRESSANTS- Tricyclic antide- pressants	Amitriptyline Desipramine Doxepin Imipramine Nortriptyline Protriptyline	Methylphenidate	Methylphenidate appears to inhibit the metabolism of tricyclic antidepressants and may increase their blood levels appreciably. Paradoxically, enhanced therapeutic response may be the only observed clinical effect.	25, 26, 141, 414, 424
		Ascorbic acid	These agents tend to acidify the urine, resulting in an increased proportion of ionized drug. Thus, tubular reabsorption of the tricyclic antidepressant is decreased. This may be important in patients with hepatic malfunction in whom renal excretion of the antidepressant may assume a more important role. However, in the patient with normal hepatic function, fluctuations in **urinary pH would probably have little clinical effect.**	52, 155, 162,279, 362, 410
		Barbiturates	A. With Therapeutic Doses of Tricyclic Antidepressant: Barbiturates appear to stimulate the metabolism of tricyclic antidepressants, and may decrease their blood levels. B. With Toxic Doses of Tricyclic Antidepressant: Barbiturates may potentiate the adverse effects of toxic doses of tricyclic antidepressants (e.g., respiratory depression). It is possible that they are both competing for the same hydroxylating enzymes. Barbiturates should probably not be used in patients with tricyclic antidepressant toxicity.	14, 60, 66, 322
		Ethanol	Tricyclic antidepressants and ethanol have - combined effects on the CNS which may produce unexpected effects. The exact mechanisms are not known. Combined effects on the liver and gastrointestinal tract may also account for adverse drug interactions with ethanol and tricyclic antidepressants.	239, 255

TABLE 18. (cont'd)

Drug Class	Measured Drug	Interacting Drug	Effect	Reference
		Anticoagulants	Nortriptyline (Aventyl) appears to impair the metabolism of dicumarol, thus increasing dicumarol plasma levels and half-lives, leading to hypo prothrombinemic effect of dicumarol.	396
		Phenylbutazone	Desipramine appears to inhibit the gastrointestinal absorption of phenylbutazone. Preliminary sutdy in four subjects indicates that peak plasma phenylbutazone levels can be considerably delayed by the prior administration of desipramine. However, total phenylbutazone absorption (based on urinary excretion of oxyphenbutazone) did not appear to be affected. Thus, under the conditions of multiple dosing of phenylbutazone, this interaction may not produce clinically detectable impairment of phenylbutazone effect.	100
		Sympathominetics	The ability of tricyclic antidepressants to inhibit uptake of norepiniphrine by the adrenergic neuron may be responsible for increased responses to sympathomimetics which may occur. Although amphetamine abuse in patients on tricyclic antidepressant therapy reportedly may be fatal, case reports of such an effect appear to be lacking.	200, 324 372
		Anticonvulasants	Tricyclic antidepressants may produce epileptiform seizures in susceptible patients, expecially if large doses are used. High doses may produce grand mal seizures even in non-epileptic patients. Factors which may predispose patients to tricyclic antidepressant-induced epileptic seizures include family history of brain damage, cerebral arteriosclerosis, alcoholism, barbiturate withdrawal, and previous electroconvulsive therapy. Whether tricyclic antidepressants could antogonize the effect of anticonvulsants remains to be established.	370, 121, 406

TABLE 18. (cont'd)

Drug Class	Measured Drug	Interacting Drug	Effect	Reference
MONAMINE OXIDASE INHIBITORS	Pargyline Tranylcypromine	Meperidine	Concomitant administration of these agents may produce severe reactions including hypertension, sweating, or hypotension.	69, 397
ANTIARRHYTHMICS	Quinidine	Soldium bicarbonate Thiazide diuretics	These agents tend to render the urine alkaline, resulting in an increased proportion of un-ionized quinidine. Thus, renal tubular reabsorption of quinidine is increased and serum levels may be increased. It should also be remembered that both thiazides and parenteral quinidine tend to lower blood pressure; additive effects may be seen.	145, 217
		Coumarin	Quinidine may produce additive hypoprothrombinemic effects with coumarin anticoagulants. Theoretically, the same effect would be seen with the inandione oral anticoagulants.	142, 218
		Phenothiazines	Phenothiazines have a quinidine-like depressant action on the heart. Additive cardiac depressant effects are possible with concomitant quinidine and phenothiazine administration. It is likely that the interaction is significant. Therefore, phenothiazine-induced ventricular tachycardia should not be treated with quinidine; it should be treated much the same as is quinidine toxicity.	135, 154, 287, 352
		Propranolol	Both quinidine and propranolol exert a negative inotropic action on the heart. Due to the possibility of combined cardiac depressant effects, caution has been recommended in concurrent use of quinidine and propranolol. However, recent studies in animals have indicated that the negative inotropic effect of these two drugs, when used together, is less than one would expect on an additive basis.	121, 370
	Procainamide	Lidocaine	Not extablished. It is possible that additive neurologic side effects may be seen with concomitant use of lidocaine and procainamide.	189

TABLE 18. (cont'd)

Drug Class	Measured Drug	Interacting Drug	Effect	Reference
		Acetazolamide Sodium Bicarbonate	Not established. The limited clinical evidence available to date indicates that procainamide undergoes pH-dependent urinary excretion. Since these agents tend to increase urine pH, the possibility exists that they may affect urinary excretion, and thus, blood levels of procainamide.	407
	Propranolol	Digitalis Glycosides	Although propranolol is used in treatment of digitalis-induced arrhythmias, bradycardia due to digitalis may be potentiated by propranolol. The adverse effect was felt to represent increased sensitivity to the action of propranolol.	
		Antidiabetic Agents	A mechanism for the hypoglycemic tendency of propranolol has not been established, although it has been proposed that propranolol interferes with catecholamine-induced glycogenolysis. Beta-adrenergic blockade does appear to reduce the rise in blood glucose following epinephrine injection. Although the mechanism is undetermined, it is well established that propranolol blunts the rebound of blood glucose following insulin-induced hypoglycemia. This effect would presumably also occur following the use of oral hypoglycemics. The possibility that propranolol may prevent the signs of hypoglycemia (e.g., glycemia (e.g., sweating,tachycardia) increases the importance of this interaction.	2, 19, 37 225
		Phenothiazines	Phenothiazines and β-adreneric blocking agents, such as propranolol may have additive hypotensive effects, the mechanisms of which have not been fully established. However, it is likely that high doses of phenothiazine compounds would be necessary before these additive hypotensive effects would casue clinical concern.	38

TABLE 18. (cont'd)

Drug Class	Measured Drug	Interacting Drug	Effect	Reference
ANTICOAGULANTS		Acetaminophen	One study in which acetaminophen (2.6 Gm/day for 2 weeks) was given to patients on various oral anticoagulants demonstrated a mean increase of 3.7 seconds in the prothrombin time as compared to a placebo. A subsequent study found acetaminophen (3 Gm/day for 2 weeks) to have no effect on the prothrombin time of response to warfarin. Others found 2 doses of 650 mg of acetaminophen to have no effect on the prothrombin time response to oral anticoagulants. From available evidence, therapeutic doses of acetaminophen appear to produce slight, if any, increase in the hypoprothrombinemic response.	27, 29, 389
		Ethanol	1. The mechanism by which ethanol enhances the effect of oral anticoagulants has not been established. 2. The increase in warfarin metabolism in heavy drinkers is probably due to ethanol-induced stimulation of hepatic microsomal enzymes.	23, 125, 359
		Chloramphenicol	1. Chloramphenicol may decrease vitamin K produced by gut bacteria; a hypoprothrombinemic effect due to an action within the hepatic cell may also be involved. 2. Chloramphenical has also been shown to inhibit the metabolism of bishydroxycoumarin, perhaps by inhibiting hepatic microsomal enzymes. The intrinsic hypoprothrombinemic activity of chloramphenicol plus its ability to markedly prolong the half-life of bishydroxy coumarin dictates extreme caution in patients receiving oral anticoagulants. Chlorphenicol produced a two-to four-fold increase in the half-life of bishydroxy-coumarin in four patients.	91, 125, 214
		Cholestyramine	1. Chlestyramine may bind warfarin in the gut and impair its absorption.	82, 83, 139, 165, 273

TABLE 18. (cont'd)

Drug Class	Measured Drug	Interacting Drug	Effect	Reference
			2. Hypoprothrombinemia with bleeding has occured in persons treated with cholestyramine in the absence of oral anticoagulants. This is presumably due to inhibition of vitamin K absorption.	
		Salicylates	Salicylates tend to reduce plasma prothrombin levels, especially if large doses are given. It is also possible that salicylates may displace coumarin anticoagulants from plasma protein binding. Other factors to consider are the gastro-intestinal bleeding which salicylates may produce and the ability of aspirin to impair primary therapeutically under carefully controlled conditions. However, most patients on oral anticoagulant therapy should probably avoid more than occasional use of small doses of aspirin. Sodium salicylate does not appear to affect platelets as does aspirin, and may be less likely to pratelets, etc.). Aspirin and oral anticoagulants have been used together oduce gastrointestinal bleeding. Thus, if a salicylate must be used, sodium salicylate is probably preferable. If a mild analgesic is needed, acetaminophen is preferable to a salicylate.	42, 96, 124, 125, 152, 389
		Tolbutamide	Tolbutamide may initially enhance the anti-coagulant effects of bishydroxycoumarin due to displacement from plasma protein binding, followed by antagonism of anticoagulant effect due to increased metabolism. Bishydroxycoumarin enhances the effect of tolbutamide, and it is probable that the elevated blood levels of tolbutamide increase the displacements of bishydroxycoumarin from plasma proteins.	323, 411

TABLE 18. (cont'd)

Drug Class	Measured Drug	Interacting Drug	Effect	Reference
		Barbiturates	Two factors appear to be involved. First, barbiturates may decrease gastrointestinal absorption of bishydroxycoumarin. Secondly, barbiturates appear to induce hepatic microsomal enzymes resulting in increased metabolism of coumarin anticoagulants. Phenobarbital, butabarbital, heptabarbital, secobarbital, and amobarbital have been shown to decrease the response to coumarin anticoagulants in man. Most barbiturates probably have this ability. A patient on both a barbiturate and a coumarin anticoagulant who stops taking the barbiturate runs the risk of hemorrhage if his anticoagulant dosage is not readjusted.	28, 97, 188, 264, 336, 337
		Carbamazepine	Carbamazepine appears to enhance warfarin metabolism by induction of hepatic microsomal enzymes.	171
		Meprobamate	Although meprobamate has been listed as a drug which decreases the action of oral anticoagulants, subsequent human studies have not shown any clinically significant effect, even at any special precautions are necessary with concomitant use of meprobamate and oral anticoagulants.	95, 188
	Warfarin Sodium	Drugs bound to plasma proteins: Chloral hydrate Clofibrate Diazoxide Phenytoin Indomethacin Phenylbutazone Oxyphenbutazone Salicylates Ethacrynic acid	These agents displace the anticoagulant from the protein binding site, resulting in increased prothrombin times and risk of hemorrhage.	175, 305

TABLE 18. (cont'd)

Drug Class	Measured Drug	Interacting Drug	Effect	Reference
ANTICONVULSANTS	Primidone Ethosuximide Mephenytoin	Oral contraceptives	Not established. Oral contraceptives may result in fluid retention, which in turn may precipitate seizures in epileptics. Also, it has been suggested that contraceptive steroids may impair metabolism or plasma protein binding of anticonvulsants. Animal studies have shown estrogens to affect drug metabolism. Very little is known about this interaction from a clinical standpoint. One case of possible oral contraceptive-induced exacerbation of epilepsy has been reported. Oral contraceptives with a relatively large estrogen component may be more likely to produce fluid retention. Another case has been reported in which an oral contraceptive may have resulted in anticonvulsant toxicity in a patient receiving primidone (Mysoline), ethosuximide (Zarontin), and mephenytoin (Mesantoin). Thus, the presence of absence of adverse drug interaction in this area depends upon a variety of factors such as condition of patient, type of oral contraceptive, types of anticonvulsants, etc.	98, 126, 272
	Phenytoin	Aminosalicylic acid	Not established. If PAS does have the ability to elevate blood levels, it may be only to increase blood levels of concomitantly administered isoniazid which in turn impairs phenytoin metabolism.	231, 235, 260

TABLE 18. (con'd)

Drug Class	Measured Drug	Interacting Drug	Effect	Reference
		Bishydroxycoumarin	The interrelationships of these two drugs are exceedingly complex, with several different mechanisms apparently involved. 1) Dicumarol (bishydroxycoumarin) appears to inhibit the para-hydroxylation of phenytoin (DPH) in the liver. 2) DPH may stimulate the metabolism of dicumarol due to enzyme induction. 3) DPH may have the ability to displace dicumarol from plasma protein binding. The overall effect of these (and perhaps other) mechanisms on half-lives, blood levels, and therapeutic effect of the two drugs will require much more study. On the basis of current knowledge, the following clinical effects may be expected: 1. If dicumarol is given to a patient maintained on DPH: a) Serum levels of DPH are likely to increase, perhaps to a point where signs of DPH intoxication occur; b) Higher than normal doses of dicumarol might be required, but this has not yet been documented clinically. 2. If DPH is given to a patient maintained on dicumarol: a) A transient initial increase in anticoagulant effect due to displacement of dicumarol might take place. (This has not yet been documented clinically). b) A decrease in anticoagulant effect might take place, possibly due to enzyme induction, which occurs within a week or two of initiation of DPH therapy.	172, 173, 260, 339

TABLE 18. (Cont'd)

Drug Class	Measured Drug	Interacting Drug	Effect	Reference
		Chloramphenicol	Chloramphenicol appears to inhibit the metabolism of phenytoin by affecting microsomal enzyme activity in the liver. Although only a few patients have been involved in the study of this interaction, evidence available strongly indicates that it does occur. Serum levels of DPH rise considerably and about a twofold increase in the half-life was observed.	212, 298, 299
		Disulfiram	Disulfiram appears to inhibit the metabolism of phenytoin in the liver. Blood levels of phenytoin are increased and urinary excretion of the major metabolite (HPPH) is decreased. Disulfiram (400 mg/day) has been shown to considerably increase serum phenytoin (DPH) concentrations in several patients. The effect was rapid, with increases in serum DPH occurring within four hours of the administration of the first dose of disulfiram. The effect was also prolonged, requiring about three weeks to insure that phenytoin levels had returned to normal. Many of the patients were also taking other drugs, however, and it would be desirable to study patients receiving only disulfiram and phenytoin to confirm these findings.	
		Isoniazid	Isoniazid appears to inhibit the metabolism of phenytoin in the liver. Blood levels of phenytoin are	65, 231, 232 235, 290

TABLE 18. (cont'd)

Drug Class	Measured Drug	Interacting Drug	Effect	Reference
			increased and urinary excretion of the major metabolite (HPPH) is decreased. Administration of INH alone as well as in combination with aminosalicylic acid in patients receiving phenytoin has been shown to result in signs of phenytoin intoxication. This interaction is probably most important in patients who are "slow" metabolizers of INH, and in those receiving both INH and PAS. In both cases, INH blood levels tend to be higher.	
		Salicylates	Salicylates may displace phenytoin (DPH) from plasma protein binding, thus increasing the concentration of free (active) DPH in the plasma.	263, 385
		Sulfonamides	Sulfaphenazole (Sulfabid) reportedly inhibits the metabolism of phenytoin (DPH). Although this interaction apparently has been noted in patients, descriptions of the specific magnitude and incidence have not appeared. Another sulfonamide, sulfisoxazole (Gantrisin), has been shown to displace DPH from plasma protein binding in vitro.	172, 260, 263
		Carbamazepine	Carbamazepine appears to enhance phenytoin (DPH) metabolism by induction of hepatic microsomal enzymes. In a preliminary study, carbamazepine appeared to decrease serum DPH levels in three of seven patients. In addition, all of five patients manifested decreases in DPH	

TABLE 18. (cont'd)

Drug Class	Measured Drug	Interacting Drug	Effect	Reference
			half-life from an intravenous dose of DPH before and during carbamazepine therapy (600 mg daily).	
		Folic acid	Replacement of folic acid in folate-deficient patients receiving phenytoin (DPH) may increase the metabolism of DPH with a resultant decrease in serum DPH levels.	46, 62, 185, 197
		Phenobarbital	Phenobarbital administration results in induction of hepatic microsomal enzymes, with resultant increase in phenytoin (DPH) metabolism. However, phenobarbital also appears to competitively inhibit the metabolism of phenytoin. With normal doses of phenobarbital, the enzyme induction would occur, but the competitive inhibition would be negligible. Large doses of phenobarbital, and perhaps normal doses in patients with impaired liver function, may elevate serum phenytoin levels. Epileptic patients who manifest decreases in phenytoin blood levels due to phenobarbital do not appear to be adversely affected clinically and no action is required. Some patients receiving DPH as an antiarrhythmic might manifest clinically significant decreases in serum DPH, but this remains to be shown clinically. Large doses of phenobarbital should probably be avoided in patients with high blood levels of phenytoin, especially if signs of intoxication are present.	73, 105, 140 222, 233, 234

TABLE 18. (cont'd)

Drug Class	Measured Drug	Interacting Drug	Effect	Reference
ANTIBIOTICS	Aminosalicylic acid	Isoniazid	Patients maintained on DPH and a barbiturate should be observed for signs of DPH intoxication if the barbiturate therapy is stopped. Aminosalicylic acid reduces the acetylation of isoniazid, resulting in increased INH blood levels. This interaction is generally considered beneficial rather than harmful. The incidence of excessive blood levels of isoniazid due to aminosalicylic acid therapy is probably quite low.	156
		Salicylates	Not established. Aminosalicylic acid is not similar to the salicylates pharmacologically and apparently does not produce salicylism. An effect of salicylates on the renal excretion or plasma protein binding of PAS may be involved.	21, 156
	Cephalosporins	Gentamicin	Gentamicin and cephalosporins may have additive nephrotoxic effects. Preliminary clinical observation in 15 patients indicates that gentamicin plus cephalosporins may result in nephrotoxicity.	57, 78, 304
	Furazolidone	Tricyclic antidepressants	A single case has appeared in which a patient receiving amitriptyline (Elavil) developed a toxic psychosis soon after furazolidone therapy was begun. However, other drugs were being taken, and it was not established that drug interaction was responsible.	5
	Griseofulvin	Barbiturates	Earlier reports indicated that phenobarbital may increase the metabolism of griseofulvin by hepatic microsomal enzyme induction. However, more recent evidence	77, 332, 379

TABLE 18. (cont'd)

Drug Class	Measured Drug	Interacting Drug	Effect	Reference
	Isoniazid	Ethanol	from pharmacokinetic studies has shown that phenobarbital impairs the absorption of griseofulvin. Chronic alcoholics reportedly metabolize isoniazid more rapidly than nonalcoholics	275
		Rifampin	There is some clinical evidence to indicate that the combined use of INH and rifampin may result in hepatotoxicity, especially in patients with previous liver impairment and/or in those who are slow INH inactivators. There is also reported evidence that rifampin half-life may be reduced in the presence of INH.	20, 238
	Aminoglycosides	Combined Use of Two or More Aminoglycoside Antibiotics	The combined or sequential use of aminoglycoside antibiotics increases the chance of ototoxicity and nephrotoxicity.	199, 348
	Methenamine	Sulfonamides	1. With some sulfonamides the danger of crystalluria is enhanced in the presence of an acid urine. Methenamine requires a urine pH of about 5.5 or less in order to be active. 2. The concomitant administration of methenamine compounds and sulfamethizole frequently results in formation of a precipitate in the urine. Methenamine and sulfathiazole reportedly result in a similar effect.	405
	Penicillins	Neomycin	In one study of five volunteers, neomycin (3.0 Gm 4/day) reduced serum concentrations of penicillin V by over 50% as compared to control values. It is possible that penicillin G would be similarly affected.	89

TABLE 18. (cont'd)

Drug Class	Measured Drug	Interacting Drug	Effect	Reference
	Sulfonamides	Sulfinpyrazone	Sulfinpyrazone may displace some sulfonamides from plasma protein binding, resulting in more active (free) drug in the plasma. An effect on the renal excretion may also be involved.	30, 143
	Sulfonamides	Indomethacin Phenylbutazone Salicylates	These drugs reportedly increase sulfonamide blood levels. In cases of altered distribution and excretion of sulfonamides clinical significance would be dependent upon a number of variables, such as: 1. Extent of protein binding of the specific sulfonamide in queston. 2. Whether the sulfonamide was being used to treat a urinary tract infection or some other infection. 3. Plasma albumin level of patient. 4. Number and type of other drugs being administered. 5. Doses of drugs involved.	14, 30
		Barbiturates	It has been proposed that sulfisoxazole competes with thiopental for plasma protein binding. In one study involving 48 patients, intravenous sulfisoxazole reduced the amount of thiopental required for anesthesia and shortened the awakening time.	103, 104
	Tetracyclines	Antacids	Antacids containing divalent or trivalent cations (e.g., calcium, magnesium, aluminum) impair the absorption of orally administered tetracyclines. This effect has been attribued to chelation of the cation by the tetracycline.	41, 347, 359

TABLE 18. (cont'd)

Drug Class	Measured Drug	Interacting Drug	Effect	Reference
ANTINEOPLASTICS	Methotrexate	Phenytoin	Phenytoin reportedly may displace methotrexate from plasma protein binding, thus enhancing its effect.	178
	Methotrexate	Salicylates	Salicylates have been shown to displace methotrexate from plasma protein binding, resulting in an increase in free methotrexate. Also, methotrexate undergoes renal tubular secretion which appears to be blocked by salicylates.	116, 253
		Sulfonamides	Studies on man have shown sulfisoxazole infusions to decrease plasma protein-bound methotrexate by about one fourth. Sulfisoxazole may also have a minor inhibitory effect on the renal tubular secretion of methotrexate.	240, 253
MONOAMINE OXIDASE INHIBITORS(MAO)	Tranylcypromine Trifluoperazine	Phenothiazines	Increased side effects of the phenothiazines (e.g., extrapyramidal reactions) reportedly may occur with concomitant use of MAO and phenothiazines. In at least one of these (using tranylcypromine and trifluoperazine), side effects of both agents were reportedly decreased by using them in combination. It has also been proposed that trifluoperazine protects against tyramine-induced hypertensive crises in patients receiving tranylcypromine.	181, 363
	(Ibid)	Tricyclic antidepressants	Severe reactions have been reported with the concomitant administration of an MAO inhibitor and a tricyclic antidepressant.	354, 363, 417

TABLE 18. (cont'd)

Drug Class	Measured Drug	Interacting Drug	Effect	Reference
			However, there is increasing evidence that MAOI and tricyclic antidepressants can be given safely together in most patients if the following precautions are used: 1. Avoiding large doses 2. Giving the drugs orally 3. Avoiding tranylcypromine 4. Avoiding imipramine 5. Monitoring the patient closely	
MISCELLANEOUS DRUG-DRUG INTER-ACTIONS	Ethanol	Salicylates	Ethanol appears to increase the gastrointestinal bleeding produced by salicylates.	40, 61, 118, 159, 289, 418
		Central nervous system depressants	Additive effects may be seen with concomitant use of ethanol and CNS depressants.	146, 311, 338, 425
	Antacids	Phenothiazines	In one study of ten patients receiving large doses of chlorpromazine, the concomitant administration of an antacid (Aludrox) resulted in 10 to 45% decreases in urinary chlorpromazine excretion. Preliminary information from another study indicates that an antacid containing magnesium trisilicate and aluminum hydroxide may result in decreased blood levels of chlorpromazine given as an oral suspension. Thus, a decreased therapeutic response to chlorpromazine seems possible, and one possible case of this has been reported.	127, 137, 368
	Barbiturates	Antidiabetic agents	Sulfonylurea hypoglycemics (e.g., tolbutamide, chlorpropamide) reportedly may prolong the effects of barbiturates.	24, 316

TABLE 18. (cont'd)

Drug Class	Measured Drug	Interacting Drug	Effect	Reference
		Phenothiazines	Barbiturates presumably increase the metabolism of chlorpromazine by induction of hepatic microsomal enzymes. The fact that urinary excretion of the conjugated fraction of chlorpromazine is increased following phenobarbital supports this view.	107, 137
	Digitoxin	Barbiturates	Phenobarbital appears to enhance the metabolism of digitoxin to digoxin, presumably due to induction of hepatic microsomal enzymes. Decreased plasma digitoxin levels and a shortened digitoxin half-life have been demonstrated when phenobarbital is given to patients receiving digitoxin. The increased conversion of digitoxin to digoxin and other metabolites could decrease the therapeutic effect since digoxin has a much shorter half-life than digitoxin.	195, 368
		Phenytoin	Phenytoin (DPH) appears to enhance the metabolism of digitoxin, probably by induction of hepatic microsomal enzymes.	368
	Indomethacin	Salicylates	One study indicated that aspirin might impair gastrointestinal absorption of indomethacin, thus decreasing indomethacin serum levels. Subsequent study using different methods has failed to confirm the presence of drug interaction, and it appears that perhaps no clinically significant interaction occurs.	87, 198
	Lithium Carbonate	Phenothiazines	Both phenothiazines and lithium carbonate have exhibited hyperglycemic tendencies	423

TABLE 18. (cont'd)

Drug Class	Measured Drug	Interacting Drug	Effect	Reference
		Sodium Chloride	The excretion of lithium appears to be proportional to the intake of sodium chloride. Patients on salt-free diets who receive lithium carbonate are prone to the development of lithium toxicity. Large doses of sodium chloride increase lithium excretion and have been recommended by some for the treatment of lithium intoxication.	54, 321
	Salicylates	Phenylbutazone	Phenylbutazone inhibits the urico-suria which usually follows large doses of salicylates. It is also possible that salicylates compete with phenylbutazone for plasma protein bindings.	56, 308
	Methotrexate	Leucovorin	Administration of leucovorin immediately (2 hours) following methotrexate infusions will de-crease the toxicity effect associated with methotrexate therapy. Simulta-neous administration of these two agents will reduce the efficacy of methotrexate.	117, 244

6.   Measurement Techniques

Knowledge of the analytical systems used for the measurement of a drug level may be important for the interpretation of same. For example, clinical laboratories have frequently used fluorometric methods for the determination of plasma concentration of quinidine, which are essentially nonspecific and may measure not only the plasma quinidine concentration, but also dihydroquinidine (an impurity in the manufacture of quinidine), and the metabolites of quinidine, 3-hydroxyquinidine and 2'-oxoquinidinone. Improvements in assay techniques have led to a wide array of methods which impart various degrees of sensitivity and specificity—extractions which remove impurities, or which remove metabolites but not the impurity, homogenous enzyme immunoassay technique, and liquid chromatography, which has been proven to be highly specific. The reported therapeutic ranges for each laboratory may vary greatly, and for this reason it is important to know the method of assay, before clinical interpretation can be fully undertaken. For example, the Cramer-Isaksson double-extraction fluorometric assay method for quinidine has been reported to give a therapeutic range of 2.3-5.0 mg/liter, while the published HPLC therapeutic levels have been as much as 50% less.

Specific criteria for each system of analysis must be adhered to by each laboratory performing drug monitoring in order to develop the necessary analytical proficiency necessary to provide reliable plasma/serum levels. While developing many of the analytical schemes and assay systems, we have found the following set of guidelines valuable in assessing whether or not a particular analytical system can be fully used in a rigorous routine drug monitoring program:

1. Does isolation of the drug from its biologic matrix give an analytical advantage?
2. What advantage does chemical modification of the compound provide?
3. How is specificity imparted to the assay?
4. How is the mass of drug determined and how is the procedure standardized against reference materials?
5. What limits the sensitivity of the assay system?
6. What are the theoretical and practical limitations to the precision of the procedure?
7. What is the state of the art regarding automation of the procedure and data analysis?
8. What aspects of the analytical procedure must be quality controlled?
9. What are the costs for batch and stat analyses and how much time is required for each?
10. What future developments will ensure a continued role for this system of analysis?

There are several procedures available for the analysis of therapeutically monitored drugs, including colorimetric, ultra-violet spectrometry, gas-liquid chromatography, liquid chromatography and a number of immunological assays. Briefly described, the assays are as follows:

Gas-Liquid Chromatography (GLC). GLC is essentially a separation tool. In this technique a sample is carried through a column by an inert carrier gas and non-volatile solvent which is usually supported on an inert solid material. The solvent selectively retards the sample constituents, according to their distribution coefficient until they form separate "bands" in the carrier gas. These bands elute from the column in the carrier gas stream and are recorded by a detector.

Liquid Chromatography (LC or HPLC). The sample is dissolved in a suitable solvent and injected through a septum into a tube with solid particles. With the proper operating conditions and packing, the components of the sample can be separated quantitatively. These separated constituents are eluted with the solvent and measured using a suitable detector. The signal from the detector is displayed on a strip-chart and quantitized electronically.

Homogenous Enzyme Assays (EMIT). The term homogenous enzyme assay is used to distinguish the method from other immunochemical methods, which are heterogenous and depend at some stage on the physical separation of antigen bound to antibody from the unbound antibody. In the EMIT assay, an enzyme is conjugated to the drug to be assayed in such a fashion that it does not alter its activity. When this drug-enzyme conjugate is bound to the antibody for the drug, the active site of the enzyme is blocked and thus excludes the substrate and the enzyme activity is reduced. When the complex is not bound, the active site is available to interact with the substrate. If free drug is present in the unknown sample, this will bind to the antibody, thus preventing the binding of the drug-enzyme conjugate. This decreases the antibody-induced inactivation of the enzyme in proportion to the drug concentration.

Hemagglutination Inhibition (HI). In the performance of HI tests a drop of a diluted specimen is placed in a well of a microtiter plate or tube. A quantity of reconstituted antiserum is added to it, and between the antibody and the antigen contained in the specimen, a drop of fixed cells containing the same antigen being detected is added to the well. If the specimen contains the drug being tested, the antibody will be neutralized, thus permitting the cells to settle in a discrete pellet. The absence of the drug in the specimen will result in sufficient free antibody to react with the antigen on the cell or other particle. The cells will therefore not settle in a pellet and the titer tray or tube will show a completely transparent solution. One of the major assets of the HI test as compared to other immunological detection methods is the lack of elaborate and expensive equipment. The only equipment requirements are the titer trays or tubes, and Pasteur pipettes.

Radioimmunoassay (RIA). A radiolabeled substance (antigen, radioligand) binds to an antibody. Addition of unlabeled antigen results in a competition with the radioligand for binding sites, thus reducing the fraction of radioligand bound. By measuring either standard curve, the amount of antigen present in an unknown samples can then be determined.

Atomic Absorption (AA). A sample is vaporized by aspiration into a hot flame. This converts metallic elements in the sample into unexcited ground state atoms which can absorb light of specific wavelengths. This light, known as resonant radiation, is the same that would be emitted by these atoms if they were excited. Resonant radiation, produced with a hollow cathode lamp containing the measured element of interest, is passed through the sample to be analyzed. The beam enters a monocaromator set for radiation characteristic for that element, and the amount of adsorption is proportional to the concentration of the element in the sample. The signal can be traced on a strip recorder or displayed on a meter.

Mass Spectrometry (MS). Individual gas molecules are bombarded by electrons, creating a variety of ions. A portion of the ions are formed into an ion beam which is accelerated through a magnetic field. A varying accelerating voltage causes the ions to separate according to their masses so that only one species at a time reaches the detector. Each molecule has a unique cracking pattern which is characteristic of its molecular structure. When the intensities of the different ion currents are related to the masses, a mass spectrum of the drug is obtained.

Ultra-violet Spectrometry (U.V.). Electronic transitions in a given molecule give rise to specific absorption bands at definite wavelengths which can be used for the indentification and quanitation of the molecule. The intensity of absorption is a measure of the concentration of the absorbing entity present. Since, however, ultraviolet absorption bands (200 to 400 m) are, in general, broad, there can be considerable overlap for different compounds and in order to identify more postively an unknown, the wavelength and specific absorption (E 1%, 1 cm.) should be considered.

Colorimetric Analysis. Many drug substances give distinct colors when brought into contact with various chemical reagents. Many of these reactions are capable of being developed into colorimetric reactions which can be measured quantitatively (400 to 700 m) either by making visual comparison of the color of the unknown with that of solutions of known composition or by measuring the intensity of color in a spectrophotometer.

In summary, many different methods utilizing a wide variety of analytical techniques are available for therapeutically monitoring various drugs, however not a single method is capable of determining simultaneously all drugs and their metabolities. Each method varies as to the time of analysis, equipment, cost and expertise. Table 19 expresses the author's opinions on recommended analytical procedures for various drug compounds based upon literature references and "hands-on" personal experience with thousands of assays.

Table 20 compares the advantages and disadvantages, in the authors' experience, of the more commonly utilized analytical systems for therapeutic drug monitoring, especially from the point of view of production and cost. Since each laboratory should assess its workload requirements, cost constraints, spectrum of assays necessary, and other factors, including technical expertise, when developing any given drug monitoring program, the advantages and disadvantages cited may have to be modified for each laboratory.

Realizing the ramifications of over- or under-dosing a patient based on an inaccurate plasma/serum drug level determination, there can be no short-cuts to this approach. Table 19 lists the analytical criteria necessary for method development to insure analytical accuracy and reliability that we have followed in developing many successful therapeutic drug monitoring programs.

The development of drug monitoring program mandates an onus on the laboratory releaseing plasma/serum drug determinations to supply interpretative data such as the therapeutic and toxic published ranges and limits of error of assay to the medical community, not just to release numbers. Physicians, pathologists, and laboratorians must all work in close harmony, in a concerted, cooperative atmosphere. This puts a great burden on the laboratory and its staff, for continuing education and analytical proficiency.

The American Association of Clinical Chemistry's Therapeutic Drug Monitoring Continuing Education and Quality Control Program has instituted sessions and begun to bridge the gap between physician and laboratory towards understanding the many ramifications of plasma/serum drug level determinations. Salient features of this program include:

(1) Monthly distribution of quality control sera (3 vials 5 ml. each) — containing antiepileptic, antibiotic, antidepressant, antiarrhythmic, and other monitored drugs — more than 20 therapeutic drugs monitored each month.

(2) Rapid turn around time (usually within 10 days) of target values and histrograms, by analytical method and statistical summary.

(3) An active continuing education program (formal or informal) of monthly manuscripts, case-histories, and new technology.

(4) A monthly update, with an active participant and reader feedback of current problems, publications, and other pertinent comments.

Another program which has proven highly educational and served as an added quality control check for analytical determinations for therapeutic drug monitoring is the America College of American Pathologists' Therapeutic Drug Monitoring Survey. Features of this service include:

(1) Four yearly shipments, containing six sera per shipment, consisting of fourteen drugs as regular analytes.

(2) "Wild card" vials, normally in two of the yearly shipments, containing drugs not routinely included as regular drugs in the survey.

(3) Computerized summary of data analysis, reported by analytical method, with statistical summary.

(4) Educational critiques covering selected aspects of therapeutic drug monitoring.

TABLE 19. Recommended "State of the Art" Analytical Techniques for Selected Drugs

Drug		Drug/Metabolite	Recommended Method
Brand Name	Generic Name	Measured	of Analysis[1]
Amikin	Amikacin	Same	RIA; HPLC; Microbio-logical; IMF
Aspirin	Salicylate	Same	Colorimetric; HPLC
Aventyl	Nortriptyline	Same	GLC; HPLC; RIA
Celontin	Clonazepam	Same	GLC; HPLC
Clonopin	Methsuximide	Same	GLC; HPLC
		Normethsuximide	EMIT(Normethsuximide)
Dalmane	Flurazepam	Same	GLC; HPLC
		N-desalkyl-flurazepam	
Depakene	Valproic acid	Same	GLC; HPLC; EMIT
Dilantin	Phenytoin	Same	HPLC; EMIT; GLC; RIA; IMF
Dimethadione	Dimethadione	Same	GLC; HPLC
Doriden	Glutethimide	Same	GLC; HPLC
Elavil	Amitriptyline	Same	GLC; HPLC; RIA
		Nortriptyline	
Elixophyllin	Theophylline	Same	HPLC; EMIT; GLC; IMF
Eskabarb	Phenobarbital	Same	HPLC; EMIT; GLC; RIA
Eskalith	Lithium		AA
Garamycin	Gentamicin	Same	RIA; HPLC; Microbio-logical; HI ; IMF
Haldol	Haloperidol	Same	GLC
Inderol	Propranolol	Same	HPLC; Fluoro-metric; GLC
		4-hydroxypropranolol	
INH	Isoniazid	Same	GLC
Lanoxin	Digoxin	Same	RIA; EMIT
Librium	Chlordiazepoxide	Same	GLC; HPLC
		Desmethylchlordia-zepoxide	
		Demoxepam	
Mebaral	Mephobarbital	Same	GLC; EMIT; HPLC
		Phenobarbital	
Mellaril	Thioridazine	Same	GLC; HPLC
		Mesoridazine	
Mesantoin	Mephenytoin	5-ethyl-5-phenyl-hydantoin	GLC; HPLC
Milontin	Phensuximide	Same	GLC; HPLC
Mysoline	Primidone	Same	HPLC; EMIT; GLC
		Phenobarbital	
		Phenylethyl-malonamide	
Nebcin	Tobramycin	Same	RIA; HPLC; Microbio-logical; IMF

TABLE 19 (cont.)

Drug Brand Name	Drug Generic Name	Drug/Metabolite Measured	Recommended Method of Analysis
Norpace	Disopyramide	Same	HPLC; GLC; EMIT
Norpramin	Desipramine	Same	GLC; HPLC; RIA
Orinase	Tolbutamide	Same	GLC; HPLC
Paradione	Paramethadione	Same	GLC; HPLC
		5-ethyl-5-methyl-2, 4-oxazolidine-dione	
Peganone	Ethotoin	Same	GLC; HPLC
Pronestyl	Procainamide	Same N-acetyl-procainamide	HPLC; EMIT;
Quinidex	Quinidine	Same	Fluorometric; HPLC; EMIT
Sinequan	Doxepin	Same Nordoxepin	GLC; HPLC: RIA
Solganal	Gold Salts	Same	AA
Tegretol	Carbamazepine	Same Carbamazepine-10, 11 epoxide	HPLC; EMIT; GLC
Thorazine	Chlorpromazine	Same	GLC; HPLC
Tofranil	Imipramine	Same Desipramine	GLC; HPLC; RIA
Tranxene	Clorazepate	Nordiazepam	GLC; HPLC
Tridione	Trimethadione	Same Dimethadione	GLC; HPLC
Tylenol	Acetaminophen	Same	Colorimetric; GLC; HPLC
Valium	Diazepam	Same Desmethyldiazepam	GLC; HPLC
Xylocaine	Lidocaine	Same Monoethylglycine-xylidide	GLC; EMIT; HPLC
Zarontin	Ethosuximide	Same	HPLC; GLC; EMIT

[1]GLC: Gas liquid chromatography; HPLC: High performance liquid chromatography; RIA: Radioimmunassay; AA: Atomic absorption; EMIT: Homogenous enzyme immunoassay; HI: Hemagglutination inhibition; IMF: Immunofluorescence.

TABLE 20. Analytical Systems for Drug Monitoring

UV — VIS

ADVANTAGES	DISADVANTAGES
	Relatively Large Sample Size
Low Reagent Cost	Sample Preparation
	Interferences
Low Equipment Cost	Non-Specificity
	Sample Through-Put
Stats	Sensitivity
	Not Versatile

IMMUNOFLUORESCENCE

ADVANTAGES	DISADVANTAGES
Small Sample	
Moderate Equipment Cost	
Minimum Training Time	High Reagent Cost
No Shelf-Life Problems	One Reagent Source
Stats	Not Versatile
Limited Sample Preparation	Linearity
Multiple Assays Per System	
Automation	

RADIO-IMMUNO ASSAY

ADVANTAGES	DISADVANTAGES
	Sample Pretreatment
Small Sample	Limit Shelf-Life
Stats	Mod. To High Equipment Cost
Multiple Assays Per System	One Reagent Source
Linearity	High Reagent Cost
Automation	Not Versatile
Sensitive Therapeutic Range	Moderate Training Time
	Radioactive Material

ENZYME-AUGMENTED ASSAY[1]

ADVANTAGES	DISADVANTAGES
No Sample Preparation	
Small Sample	Very High Reagent Cost
Moderate Equipment Cost	One Reagent Source
Minimum Training Time	Not Versatile
Stats	Linearity
Minimum Down Time	
Automation	

GLC

ADVANTAGES	DISADVANTAGES
	Sample Pretreatment
	Detectors
Versatile	Difficult To Trouble Shoot
Small Sample	Not Adaptable To Stats
Relatively Low Reagent Cost	Down Time
Moderate Equipment Cost	Leaks
	Diff. Columns
	Low Column Life

[1]Emit ® as an example.

HPLC

ADVANTAGES	DISADVANTAGES
Versatile	
Small Sample	
Relatively Low Reagent Cost	
Moderate Equipment Cost	Sample Pretreatment
Minimum Training Time	Detectors
Ease Of Trouble Shooting	Sample Through-Put
No Derivitization	
Stats	
Low Drift	
Minimum Down Time	

TABLE 21. Analytical Criteria for Therapeutic Drug Monitoring Assays

1. **Specimen:** Stability of constituent must be specified; specify complete collection procedure and patient preparation.

2. **Procedure:** Presented as a detailed, step-by-step outline with pertinent references.

3. **Quality Control Material:** Suitable material should be assayed with each run covering therapeutic and toxic ranges.

4. **Standards:** Use of aqueous standards is encouraged, based upon recovery studies, or suitable matrix utilizing a blank and at least three points.

5. **Linearity:** Complete range of assay should cover therapeutic, and if possible, toxic levels.

6. **Stability:** Stability of final measured product should be stated.

7. **Reaction Time:** The reaction time(s) or incubation time(s) over the entire therapeutic/toxic ranges should be established.

8. **Recovery Studies:** The % recovery at three levels (sub-therapeutic, therapeutic, and toxic) should be calculated.

9. **Precision:** (a) Within day precision at three levels with at least twenty-five samples; (b) Day-to-day precision at three levels over a 30-day or longer period, expressed as coefficient of variation (C.V.).

10. **Interferences:** (a) Effect of bilirubin up to 20 mg/dl, hemoglobin up to 500 mg/dl and lipemia (triglyceride concentration up to 500 mg/dl) should be evaluated; (b) Effect of various drugs and other potential interferences should be stated.

11. **Therapeutic/Toxic Values:** Whenever possible, therapeutic/toxic ranges with at least 100 samples each should be established at each laboratory.

12. **Comparison with Reference Method:** When possible, parallel assays should be undertaken with an accepted method, using at least 100 samples. The t test for paired data, correlation coefficient, linear regression, and the F test should be determined for analytic precision.

7. Antibiotic Assays

TESTING FOR MICROBIAL SUSCEPTIBILITY[1]

Antibiotic Impregnated Discs

The widespread use of antibiotics and the resultant occurrence of anti-biotic-resistant strains of microorganisms from hitherto sensitive strains has made it increasingly significant to determine the susceptibility of the etiological agents in a bacterial infection to a number of antibiotics and other anti-microbial agents.

One of the earliest methods utilized for the determination of the concentration of an antibiotic that would inhibit the growth of a pathogen is the tube dilution method. In this procedure serial dilutions of an antibiotic are made in a nutrient broth and the tubes so diluted are then inoculated with a constant amount of the pathogen. After incubation, the tube containing the lowest concentration of the antibiotic that prevents visible growth of the organism is called the minimun inhibitory concentration (MIC). This method of determin-ing the MIC gained credence because of the views widely held that a concen-tration of antibiotic or other anti-microbial agent thus determined could be directly related to the necessary blood level that would achieve a therapeutic result in an infectious state.

Tube Dilution Method

The tube dilution method for determining susceptibility requires a pure culture isolate of the organism to be tested. Because of the added time and materials needed, this method has not gained wide popularity. Furthermore, since many common infections are the result of the activity of more than one organism, the disc method of susceptibility testing reveals most readily which antibiotic or combination of antibiotics will suppress this mixed microbial flora. In addition, some correlation between the size of the inhibition zones shown by impregnated discs and the degree of inhibition zones shown by the tube dilution method has been demonstrated (Patrick et al., 1951). Thus the rapidity and ease of determination, and the low cost have made the disc method the one of choice.

Although relatively few antibiotics are administered that are monitored for drug levels during the course of therapy, the determination of a disc susceptibil-ity test has the indirect effect of recommending therapeutic blood levels as a

---

[1]The term 'susceptibility' is used with reference to microbial sensitivity in order to avoid possible confusion with patient sensitivity (allergy) to antibiotics.

result of the presumed relationship between the size of the zone of inhibition and the MIC value. The disc method therefore, or other methods of determining anti-microbial susceptibility that relate in performance to the disc test, is deserving of special consideration insofar as it affects the calculated recommendation of blood levels to suppress infectious agents.

The use of discs or pellets impregnated with antibiotcs in varying concen-centrations for determining microbial susceptibility has been described by numerous investigators (Vincent and Vincent, 1944; Bondi et al., 1947; Hoyt and Levine, 1947). Morley's (1945) proposal to dry impregnated discs so that they might be stored for extended periods of time enhanced the usefulness of this technique of determining microbial sensitivity (Fig. 4).

The worth of the disc tehnique for the clinical assessment of these antibiotics which might be effective and those that might have little or no effect has been substantiated by numerous reports. Broom et al. (1953) reported good correlation between the results of disc susceptibility testing and the clinical

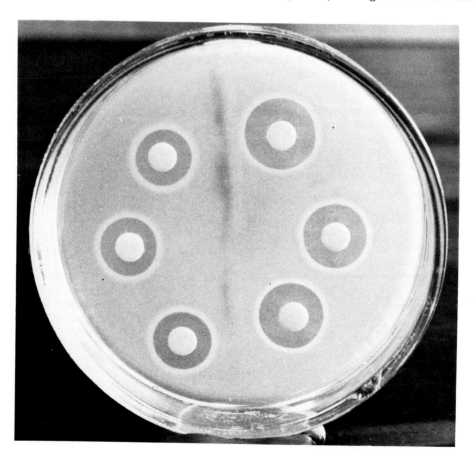

FIGURE 4. Single discs showing zones of inhibition.

course in patients with bacterial meningitis. Similar reports have also been made by other workers (Lind and Swanton, 1952; Lee, 1952).

The concept of a multi-tipped disc (Fig. 5) as well as the utilization of mechanical disc dispensers (Fig. 6) are innovations first developed and reported by Scherr(1954). Multiple-tipped discs such as the Multidisk perform as well as single discs if the drug content of the discs are the same as those of single discs (Balows and Barker, 1955; Eisenberg and Shapiro, 1958).

In many serious infections such as meningitis or in endocarditis, antimicrobial therapy will frequently have been instituted prior to the identification of the etiological agent or the determination of its antibiotic susceptibility. Specimens should be procured prior to the institution of any antibiotic therapy. It often is meaningful to perform a Gram stain on the sputum, urine or other specimen in order to provide some guide to the etiological agent, despite the fact that the demand of the time may dictate immediate institution of antibiotic

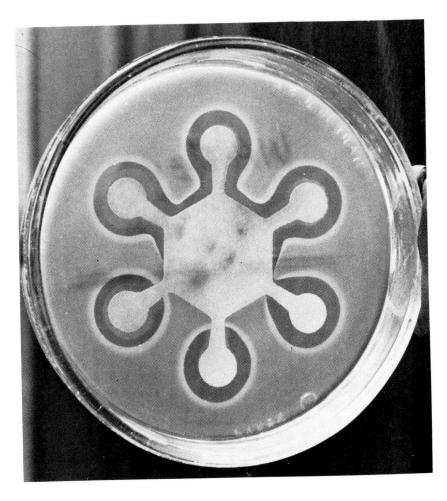

FIGURE 5 The multi-tipped disc, Multidisk, which requires no mechanical dispenser.

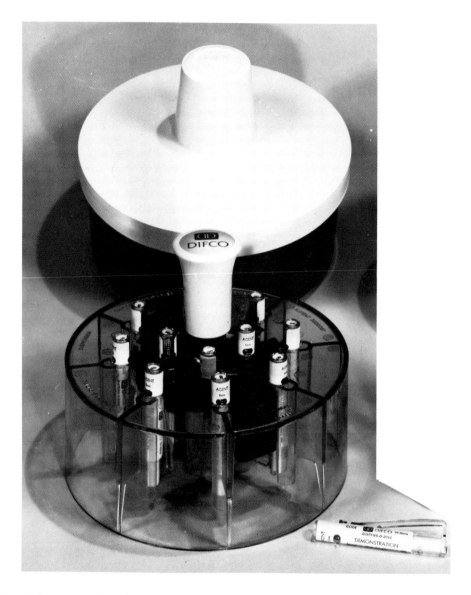

FIGURE 6. A mechanical disc dispenser for susceptibility determinations which contains as many as 12 different antimicrobial agents. Courtesy Difco Laboratories, Detroit, Michigan.

therapy. The salient advantage of susceptibility testing would be to determine if the organism is resistant to the antibiotic whose use had initially been instituted and/or the alternative antibiotics that could be utilized in the event that they may be required.

The size of the zone of inhibition is influenced by numerous factors and it is the size of the zone of inhibition from which determinations of minimum inhibitory concentrations (MIC) are directly made. The size of the zone (diameter) is determined by the concentration of the antibiotic that arrives at a position in the boundary outward from the disc where a critical population size of the organism has been reached which prevents further inhibition. If the generation time of the strain of organism being examined is short, then the critical population of numbers of bacteria will occur sooner (as contrasted with organisms having a longer generation time); the size of the zone will thereby be decreased. If the antibiotic is a relatively large molecule, then its rate of diffusion in the agar would be diminished, also resulting in a reduced zone of inhibition.

The generation time of any microorganism is markedly influenced by the temperature of incubation. It is easily shown that utilizing a generation time of 20 minutes, two cultures of the same organism, one incubated at 37° C and the other at 38°C would differ in numbers of organisms as a result of the increase in generation time. The higher temperature after three hours of incubation would account for a difference which would significantly decrease the diameter of the zone of inhibition (Garret and Wright, 1967).

An excellent study correlating the size of the zone of inhibition in a single disc test with the MIC was performed by Kanazawa (1961). Kanazawa utilized single discs from which MIC concentrations were calculated by means of standard curves; standard curves having been constructed by the utilization of 84 strains of test organisms in experiments each of which were repeated 7 times. The relationships found between the diameter of the zone of inhibition of a disc and the minimum inhibitory concentrations was further assessed in terms of the clinical course of patients whose prognosis was followed along with the determination of MIC values. The authors concluded that *"To a certain extent, a continous correlation was observed between the MIC and the clinical responses"*.[1]

In 1966 Bauer et al. correlated the disc duffusion test with the minimim inhibitory concentrations of a few hundred strains of organisms and showed that there was a relationship between the diameter of a zone of inhibition and the MIC value so determined. This led to a wider acceptance of disc sensitivity testing which method currently bears the name "Bauer-Kirby".[2] The Bauer-Kirby method as currently practiced (Federal Register 1972, 1973;) and the agar-overlay method of Barry et al. (1970) are essentially the two agar diffusion procedures principally used today.

Although the MIC values provide some semblance of standardization for the determination of the presumable effectiveness of an antibiotic against an isolated pathogen, precise information concerning the drug levels that will take place in various organs such as the lung, blood, or kidney, can only be assessed by direct assay using biological material such as spinal fluid, blood, or urine. The fact that many drugs may concentrate in the urine and therby achieve very high levels therin, could be misleading in the treatment of an infection which

---

[1]Italics our own.
[2]There is not as of this writing a consensus whether the method should be called "Bauer-Kirby" or "Kirby-Bauer", the literature being divided between both preferences.

may be present in a site other than that of the urinary tract. In general, one may operate on the basis of the fact that the serum levels that are desirable for the inhibition of an infectious state are usually considerably higher (2-4x) than the MIC values determined either directly or extrapolated from the sizes of the zones of inhibition in a disc test.

Urinary excretion is the principal route of elimination for most antimicrobial agents; where utilization of certain antibiotics such as the aminoglycosides may result in dangerously high concentrations in the blood stream of a patient who may have impaired urinary excretion, blood monitoring of the levels of such antibiotics is mandatory in order to avoid renal damage. This result has also been shown to occur with streptomycin where impaired renal function may subsequently result in ototoxicity unless careful monitoring of blood levels is performed (Carr et al., 1950).

Kit methods have been developed for determining blood levels for many of the aminoglycocides and are available for laboratory use either by radioimmunoassay, enzyme augmented assay, microbial assay, fluorescent immunoassay, or hemagglutination inhibition assay.

The Relationship Between the Zone of Inhibition and the Minimal Inhibitory Concentration (M.I.C.)

Standardization of the manufacture of susceptibility discs by the U. S. Food and Drug Administration and regulatory agencies of other countries has had the effect of insuring that, within acceptable limits, discs (or other mechanisms for performing bacterial susceptibility testing which equate to disc performance) will result in similar determinations if the same test on the same organism is performed in a number of different laboratories. This confidence unfortunately has been extrapolated also to mean that the MIC determined from the size of the zone of inhibition is a reproducible factor when different strains of microorganisms are tested against the same concentration of antibiotic-containing disc on the same Mueller-Hinton medium. The fact that this is not so is well documented by reports such as those of Trainer (1963). The relationship between the disc susceptibility testing and the tube test (MIC values) can reveal "widely varying degree of correlation depending upon the nature of the organism . . .". For example, (Trainer, 1963), 25 strains of *Pseudomonas* examined at varying concentrations in a tube dilution test and compared on six different media using both 5 μg and 30 μg sensitivity discs containing kanamycin showed the following kinds of discrepancies: eight percent of the *Pseudomonas* strains tested at 12.5 μg/ml in a tube test were considered sensitive as was 8% of the *Pseudomonas* strains tested shown to be sensitive on Mueller-Hinton medium, but at a concentration of 50 μg/ml, 72% of the same *Pseudomonas* strains were shown to be sensitive in a tube dilution test, but only 24% were considered sensitive utilizing the 5 μg disc test. Similarly, 25 strains of *Pseudomonas* tested for sensitivity to Tetracycline, both in a tube and in a disc test resulted 4% showing sensitivity in a tube test at 3.13 μg/ml concentration of tetracycline and the same 4% were also shown to be sensitive on Mueller-Hinton medium utilizing a 5 μg disc. However, at the level of 25 μg/ml in a tube test 88% were shown to be sensitive but still only 24% were sensitive at the disc test. Although these discrepancies were not found to be the rule, their occurrence was sufficiently common to warrant the admonishment that the size of the zone of inhibition, when ultimately calculated in terms of MIC, should be utilized as a guide to therapy only in the presence of other concomitant clinical findings. The relationship between the MIC determined *in vitro* and the blood levels necessary to result in inhibition of the infectious organism has some validity, but it is not because the blood levels determined in a patient can be equated directly with the MIC determined in a test tube since most microbial infections are infections of tissues. In addition, factors of diffusion in the tissues by the antibiotic, the severity of the particular infection, and other physiological conditions of the patient will necessarily result in altering the direct relationship between the MIC and the necessary blood levels required to achieve therapy of the infectious state.

Because of the laborious nature of performing tube dilution tests, and because a single mutant organism, or contaminant overgrowing a tube containing an antibiotic would result in a false negative test, disc susceptibility testing has become the one most usually practiced. The disc test relates the size of the zone of inhibition to the MIC that one would expect to find in a tube dilution test, depending upon the rigor expended for the many variables in performing the test which include:

(a)   The use of a fixed volume of Mueller-Hinton medium (with or without blood) in a Petri dish poured on a level surface.

(b)   Discs containing a concentration of an antimicrobial agent which assays in accord with government regulations.

(c)   A standardized inoculum.

The criterion (b) above deserves comment. For example, the regulations pertinent to disc testing in Canada stipulate that the concentration of antibiotic in a disc meet the labeled requirements within certain limits of assay whereas discs prepared and sold in the United States may contain very wide deviations from the labeled potency on the disc as long as they *perform as if they contained the labeled potency* in relation to standard discs, plus or minus 67% to 150% of such "labeled" potency.

Mueller-Hinton has become the recommened medium for disc susceptibility testing. This medium has a very low concentration of para-amino benzoic acid which would otherwise interfere with determinations for sulfonamide susceptibility. However, it is quite clear from the data reported by Trainer (1963) that the reason Mueller-Hinton medium results in a relatively high number of strains sensitive to antibiotics is due to the fact that it is to be considered a relatively poor medium for sustaining microbial growth of many pathogens. *The richer the medium and the more luxuriant the growth, then the lower the number of sensitive strains that may be detected.* Thus, the difference between using blood agar for determining the sensitivity to discs of kanamycin with 25 strains of *Pseudomonas* and using Mueller-Hinton medium with the some strains and the identical concentration of kanamycin discs, result in zero organisms shown to be sensitive on blood agar medium against 24% of the organisms being shown to be sensitive on Mueller-Hinton (Table 4 from Trainer's (1963) paper). Recent literature from a manufacturer of bacteriological media has been promoting an "improved" Mueller-Hinton Medium II and indicating that this new improved medium will give zones of inhibition where competitive Mueller-Hinton media would not. If two different sources of this medium can be utilized, where one will show zones of inhibition with and antimicrobial agent and the other will not, then the standardization hitherto anticipated for this method of computing MIC values falls even more by the wayside!

It has been pointed out (Gould, 1960) that infectious agents present in the tissues of a patient being treated with an antibiotic might, in fact, be more senstive to that antibiotic than would be indicated by an *in vitro* test. These results would be expected because any bacterial inoculum used either in a tube dilution test or in a agar diffusion disc test would be expectd to contain far more bacteria than that likely to be found in infected tissues. In addition, the *in vitro* organisms would usually start growth from the lag (resting) phase (in which state the bacteria would generally be more resistant to antibiotic activity) as contrasted with actively growing organisms which would be expected in infected tissue. Further, it would be expected that normal defense mechanisms of the host would operate concomitantly with antibiotic activity; a situation not comparable in an *in vitro* test.

The size of the zone of inhibition and the minimal inhibitory concentration extrapolated from it will vary radically with inoculum. Precise studies in which regression curves were determined for different inoculum sizes in order to determine their effect on the zone of inhibition by antibiotics have been made (Cooper *et al.*, 1958) and the size of the zone of inhibition may even be decreased to zero if the inoculum size is large enough. Despite attempts to control the inoculum size within some sort of limits as recommeded by the U. S. Food and Drug Administration and regulatory agencies in other countries such as Canada, the generation time of any particular organism will also influence the size of the zone of inhibition and there is no way to control this factor (Cooper *et al.*, 1958). Further, it has been shown by de Beer and Sherwood (1945) that varying the depth of the culture medium by as little as 1 mm could result in a significant altered zone of inhibition for Penicillin which could be translated as indicating almost two times the MIC value. Thus, any significant errors in the pouring of the depth of the medium in a plate or in the utilization of plates which have shrunk in thickness or in utilizing plates which have been poured on a surface not absolutely level may result in significant errors in the interpretation of the zone of inhibition.

One of the more unreliable aspects of the standardized disc test is the recommendation to "select four or five similar colonies" (*Code of Federal Regulations,* "Antibiotic Drugs Intended for Use in Laboratory Diagnosis of Disease, Subpart A — Susceptibility Disease," U. S. Food and Drug Administration) as one of the steps in isolating the etiological agent prior to the performance of the susceptibility test; *all of which would necessarily have to be of the identical organism* and concomitantly the etiological agent of the disease in question. The practice had been employed, and in some laboratories utilized to this day, in which the clinical specimen is streaked directly onto a medium upon which the antibiotic-impregnated discs are then placed for the determination of microbial susceptibilty. This procedure has the following advantages:

1. It does not make reliance solely on colonial morphology the entire basis for isolating the infectious agent.
2. It does not run the risk of altering the relative proportions of organisms present in the disease state which may be a most significant factor in the therapy of the disease in question.
3. It permits an isolation of the organism(s) by preferential inhibition of any mixed microbial flora by the various antibiotics utilized in the disc test. In other words, some of the antibiotics may inhibit the secondary organism present and by this method one can determine what antibiotic(s) would be more desirable to inhibit one or both organisms.
4. It conserves time in performing the test which otherwise would take an an additional eight hours.

Reeves *et al.* (1978) have pointed out that standardization of the inoculum by the Kirby-Bauer method is very tedious and time-consuming and there is even some doubt concerning its reliablility (Barry, 197A; Barry, 197B).

The influence of some of the above factors has been most succinctly assessed by Cooper and his colleagues at the University of Bristol:

"A proper understanding of the significance of critical concentration, time and population seems to us to be fundamental therefore for understanding growth and antibiotic action. The action of antibiotics in solid tissues is obviously limited by their diffusibility, but it has not, it seems to us, been realized that it is also limited by the critical population of organisms. If this be exceeded, i.e., if diffusion necessitates a critical time during which action must be achieved, then after this a thousandfold increase of antibiotic will be unable to stop further bacterial mutliplication at such a site. The essential requirement of early therapy is thus shown to be a theoretical requirement as well as a clinical observation — and this is quite apart from such considerations as the development of adaptive enzymes or resistant mutants, or the destruction of antibiotic by bacterial substances."

It is clear that any organism can be used to effect a straight line relationship between the diameter of the zone of inhibition and the MIC for a particular culture medium. However, 100 organisms of varying species and genera sensitive to penicillin may well give 100 regression curves of varying slopes, the mean of which is now recommeded as a standard regression curve for penicillin-resistant organisms. The utilization of a single regression curve for each anti-microbial agent obviously cannot apply to all organisms sensitive to that antibiotic; the failure to meet the criterion of a regression curve is particularly applicable to organisms that have a longer generation time and/or those that are highly fastidious in their growth requirements, such as most *Pseudomonas* strains and *Niesseria*. These failures to conform to the standard regression curves in the performance of the susceptibility test is a recognized problem by workers in the field and may require direct MIC determinations.

Dr. Hans Eriksen of the Karolinska Institute in Stockholm also concurs with the contention that there is a lack of credibility in utilizing a single regression curve for an antibiotic as being applicable to all species of bacteria that might be found susceptible to that antibiotic: "I also agree that the use of the same regression curve for all species introduces a certain error. This error is mainly related to the growth speed of different species and the critical density of the bacterial population" (Personal communication).

Lind and Swanton (1952) have also pointed out that the size of a zone of inhibition *per se* should not be relied upon as a guide to any arbitrary level of susceptibility ascribed to such measurement. They thus report that:

> "...sensitive organisms that gave zones of inhibition of 8 mm, 15 mm, or 25 mm, respectively, gave identical end points of growth inhibition by the tube dilution technic: this is contrary to certain claims that an organism is resistant unless a specified diameter of zone inhibition is demonstrated. Since this occurred regularly rather than infrequently and was supported by clinical response, it was felt that the interpretation of the width of the zone of inhibition by an antibiotic per se could not be relied on to divide the sensitive from the resistant organisms."

The disc test should be utilized as a relatively crude assessment which can be of some support to the physician either in his initial choice of an antimicrobial agent or where his initial choice may prove to be inadequate and it becomes necessary to seek an alternative antibiotic. It has been recognized, however, that "*in vitro* sensitivity results have little direct correlation with the dosage of treatment, the use of specific units of sensitivity of a microorganism to a particular antibiotic offers limited assistance to the physician and may at times provide misleading information." (Lind and Swanton, 1952).

The relationship between the size of a zone of inhibition utilizing an antibiotic-impregnated sensitivity disc and the efficacy of an antibiotic utilized to treat an infection are related by two other intermediary relationships which can be depicted as follows: the size of a zone of inhibition has some relationship to the minimal inhibitory concentration if we can rely on the regression curves provided for this relationship. The minimal inhibitory concentration is presumably related to the blood serum levels that can be directly assayed on a patient so treated. Serum levels are presumed to have a relationship to the efficacy of the antibiotic being utilized to treat a specific tissue infection. An excellent reference text has been published by Reeves *et al.* (1978) which sets forth the criteria and control methodology for the laboratory testing for antimicrobial susceptibility. Reeves *et al.* submit and support the thesis that: "...if of 100 laboratories testing a tetracycline-resistant *Staphylococcus* all report it as resistant and differentiate it clearly from a sensitive strain, precise universal standardization of methodology is of secondary importance." It is strongly recommended that a control organism of known sensitivity to the agents being tested be utilized in a control program in order to maintain data as to the continuous performance of the medium, discs, and general methodology utilized in antimicrobial susceptibility testing.

In order to reduce any deviations from the relationship of a zone of inhibition of a sensitivity disc and the MIC, a number of instruments have appeared on the market which measure the MIC directly. One such instrument miniaturizes the test tube in which the reaction takes place and by increasing the inoculum size in relation to the amount of substrate reduces the time of reading to approximately four hours. Utilizating a microtiter tray and an automated dispensing device, serial dilutions of the antibiotic and a fixed volume of inoculum of the suspect organism are delivered into small wells (Fig. 7). The utilization of such a serial dilution technique also make possible the determination of a minumum bacteriocidal concentration (MCB) which value might oftentime be more significant than the minimum inhibitory concentration.

An indirect measurement for MIC utilizes a monochromatic light source or laser beam (Fig. 8) and records the scattering of light through a culture of organisms isolated from a patient in which the inoculum is suspended in a medium of known concentration of an antibiotic whose effectiveness is to be tested. The way in which the light scatters through a radius emanating from the cuvette, called the differential light scattering (DLS) pattern, can be utilized to interpret the effectiveness of an antibiotic on a suspected organism. The instrument appears to have one advantage in that it will distinguish an increase in biomass of the cell as distinguished from an increase in cell number, a difference that frequently cannot be measured by conventional turbidometric or nephelometric measuring devices.

Some cells may increase in mass slightly in the presence of an antibiotic which is not lethal to them, but their lack of cell division would mark them as being resistant to an antibiotic if the measurement were performed nephelometrically but would be indicated as being susceptible if they merely enlarge but their cell division mechanism has been impaired

The anticipated capabilities of such a DLS determining system could be the more ready determination of the minumum biocidal levels as well as the possibility of quantitating the synergistic interaction between two antimicrobial drugs that might be prescribed concomitantly.

Another instrument (Fig. 9) also uses laser scattering at a fixed angle in order to measure microbial growth in the presence of a predetermined concentration of an antibiotic. The unique feature of this instrument is the utilization of impregnated paper discs which contain the antibiotics which are then eluted in a small chamber to provide the concentration of antibiotic necessary for the MIC determination. Results using this device can be read in approximately three to five hours and the light-scatter determinations are related to the MIC values.

Table 22 presents data indicating desirable serum levels with antibiotics and the recommended susceptibility disc concentrations in current use.

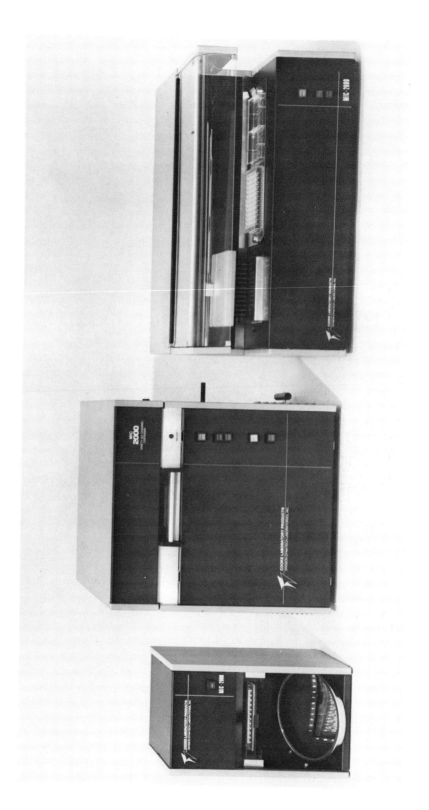

FIGURE 7. Automated dilution and dispensing device for direct measurement of MIC. Dynatech MIC-2000, courtesy of Dynatech Lab. Inc., Alexandria, Virginia.

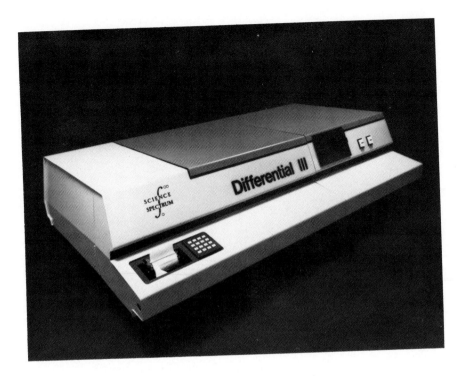

FIGURE 8. The laser operated Differential III for determining MIC values. Courtesy Science Spectrum, Santa Barbara, California.

TABLE 22. Antimicrobial Susceptibility Testing and Usual Peak Serum Levels

Antibiotic[1] (Generic name)	Trade Names	Active Content[2] in disc test[3]	Usual serum level[4] (μg/ml)
Amantadine	Symetrel®	(Not recommended)	Anti-viral agent 0.4
Amikacin	Amikin® (Bristol Labs.)	10 μg	10-25
Amoxicillin	Amoxil®, Larotid®, Polymox®, Robamox®, Trimox®, Utimox®, Wymox®	(Ampicillin class)	
Amphotericin B	Fungizone® (Squibb)	100 units	1.0
Ampicillin[5]	Alpen®, Amcill®, Ampi-Co®, Omnipen® (Wyeth), Pen A®, Penbritin® (Ayerst Labs), Pensyn®, Polycillin® (Bristol Labs), Principen®, QID amp®, SK-Ampicillin®, Supen®, Totacillin®	10μg	2.0-5.0
Bacitracin		5, 10 units	(not prescribed parenterally)
Benzanthine penicillin	Bicillin®, Permapen®	(Penicillin class)	
Capreomycin	Capastat®		15 — 50
Carbenicillin	Geocillin®, Geopen® (Roerig and Co.), Pyopen®	50,100 μg	100 — 300
Cefaclor	Ceclor®	(Cephalothin class)	15
Cefadroxil	Duricef®	(Cephalothin class)	
Cefamandole nafate	Mandol® (Eli Lilly)	30 μg	16 — 32
Cefotoxin	Mefoxin®	(Cephalothin class)	20

TABLE 22. (Cont'd)

Cephadrine	Anspor®, Velosef®	(cephalothin class)	18
Cephalexin	Keflex®	(cephalothin class)	11 — 30
Cephaloglycin	Kafocin®	(cephalothin class)	200-1300 μg/ml (urine level)
Cephaloridine	Loridine® (Eli Lilly)	(cephalothin class)	10 — 13
Cephalothin[6]	Keflin® (Eli Lilly)	30 μg	5 — 40
Cephapirin	Cefadyl®	(cephalothin class)	24
Cephazolin	Ancef®, Kefzol®	(cephalothin class)	50
Chloramphenicol	Amphicol®, Chloromycetin® (Parke-Davis)	30 μg	10.0 — 20.0
Chlortetracycline	Aureomycin® (Lederle)	10,30 μg	(same as tetracycline)
Clindamycin	Cleocin® (Upjohn)	2 μg	5.0
Cloxacillin	Tegopen® (Bristol Labs), Cloxapen®	1 μg	10.0 ± 5.0
Colistin	Coly-mycin® (Watner-Chilcott Labs)	10 μg	7.5
Cotrimoxazole	Trimethoprim and Sulphamethoxazole	1.25 μg and 23.75 μg respectively	Trimethorprim 2.0 Sulphamethoxazole 6.0
Demeclocycline	Declomycin®, Declostatin®	5 μg, 30 μg (tetracycline class)	
Dicloxacillin	Dynapen® (Bristol Labs), Pathocil®, Veracillin®	1 μg	10 ± 5
Doxycycline	Vibramycin® (Pfizer), Doxy-II®	5 μg, 30 μg	2.0 — 4.0

TABLE 22. (cont'd)

Antibiotic[1] (Generic name)	Trade Names	Active Content[2] in disc test[3]	Usual serum level[4] (μg/ml)
Erythromycin	Ilotycin® Ilosone® (Eli Lilly), Erythrocin® (Abbott), E-mycin®, Robimycin®, Pediamycin®, Wyamicin®, E.E.S.®	2 μg, 15 μg	1.0 – 2.0
Erythromycin stearate	Bristamycin®, Erypar®, Erythrocin®, Ethril®, Pfizer-E®	(Erythromycin class)	
Ethambutol	Myambutol®		4.0 – 5.0
5-Fluorocytosine	Ancobon®	(Not generally recommended)	Antifungal agent 50 – 100
Gentamicin	Geramycin® (Schering Corp.)	10 μg	2.0 – 10.0
Griseofulvin	Fulvicin®, Grifulvin V® (McNeil), Grisactin®	(not generally recommended)	1.0 – 2.0
Hetacillin	Versapen®	(Ampicillin class)	2.0 – 5.0
Isoniazid	INH, Nydrazid®, Hyzyd®, Niconyl®	(not generally recommended)	1.5 – 5.0
Kanamycin	Kantrex® (Bristol Labs)	5 μg, 30 μg	15 – 25
Lincomycin	Lincocin® (Upjohn)	(Clinamycin class)	10
Methacycline	Rhondomycin®	(Tetracycline class)	2
Methanamine mandelate	Donnasep (MP)®, Mandalay®, Mandelamine®, (Warner-Chilcott), Methavin®, Thiacide®, Trac Tab®, Uretron®, Urised®, Uristat®, Uro-Phosphate®, Uroqid-Acid®	3 mg	(urinary anti-microbial)
Methicillin[8]	Staphcillin® (Bristol Labs), Celbenin®	5 μg	20

TABLE 22. (cont'd)

Drug	Trade name (manufacturer)	Disk content	Level
Metronidazole	(for Trichomoniasis and Amebiasis)		
Miconazole	Monistat®	(not generally recommended)	5.0 (antifungal agent)
Minocycline	Minocin®, Vectrin®	(Tetracycline class)	1.0 – 3.0
Nafcillin	Nafcil®, Unipen® (Wyeth)	(represented by Methicillin)	1 – 8
Naladixic acid	NegGram® (Winthrop Labs), Wintomylon® (Winthrop Prods.)	30 μg	(urinary anti-microbial) 25 — (serum Level) 100 — 200 (urine level)
Neomycin	Mycifradin® (Upjohn), Neobiotic® (Pfizer)	30 μg	1 – 2 (poorly absorbed from gastrointetinal tract)
Nitrofurantoin	Cyantin®, Furachel®, Furadantin®, Ivadantin®, Macrodantin® (Eaton Labs), Nitrex®, Trantoin®	50, 150, 300 μg	50 – 150 (urine levels)
Nitrofurazone	Furacin®		
Novobiocin	Alkbamycin® (Upjohn)	30 μg	20
Nystatin	Mycostatin® (E.R. Squibb)	100 units	(not usually used parenterally)
Oleandomycin[9]		15 μg	0.8
Oxacillin	Bactocill®, Prostaphlin® (Bristol Labs)	(represented by Methicillin class)	10.0 ± 5.0
Oxolinic acid	Utibid® (Warner-Chilcott Labs)	2 μg	1.0 – 2.0
Oxytetracycline	Oxlopar®, Oxy-Kesso-Tetra, Oxy-Tetrachel®, Terramycin® (Pfizer)	(represented by Tetracycline)	1 – 5
Para-amino salicylic acid	Parasal®	(not generally recommended)	50 – 100

TABLE 22. (cont'd)

Antibiotic[1] (Generic name)	Trade Names	Active Content[2] in disc test[3]	Usual serum level[4] (μg/ml)
Penicillin[10]	Buffered Penicillin G, Kesso-Pen®, Pentids®, Pfizerpen G®, QID pen G®	10 units	varies widely with type of Penicillin: benzyl penicillin 10.0 penicillin V 1.0 – 3.0 procaine penicillin 1.0
Phenethicillin	Syncillin®	(represented by penicillin)	
Phenoxymethyl Penicillin (Penicillin V)	Betapen VK®, Compocillin V or VK®, Kesso-Pen VK®, Ledercillin VK®, Maxipen®, Penapar VK®, Pen-Vee-K®, Pfizerpen VK®, QID pen VK®, Robicillin VK®, SK-Penicillin VK®, Uticillin VK®, V-Cillin K®, Veetids®	(represented by Penicillin)	1.0 – 3.0
Polymyxin B	Aerosporin®	300 units	6.0 – 8.0 (1 μg = 10 units)
Rifampin	Rifadin® (Dow), Rimactane® (Ciba)	5 μg	6.0 – 8.0
Spectinomycin	Trobicin®		100
Streptomycin		10 μg	25
Sulfadiazine		300 μg	(wide variation)
Sulfamerzaine		300 μg	(wide variation)
Sulfamethoxazole	Gantanol®	300 μg	30 – 60
Sulfamethizole	Thiosulfil® (Ayerst)	250μg	
Sulfamethoxypyridazine	Kynex® (Lederle), Midicel® (Parke-Davis)	300 μg	(wide variation)

TABLE 22. (cont'd)

Drug	Brand (Manufacturer)	Disc potency	Serum level (wide variation)
Sulfathiazole		300 µg	
Sulfisoxazole	Gantrisin® (Hoffman-LaRoche)	150, 300 µg	60
Tetracycline[11]	Mysteclin-F® QID tet®, SK-Tetracycline®, Achromycin® (Lederle Labs), Achromycin V®, Achrostatin V®, Bristacycline®, Cyclopar®, Kesso-Tetra®, Panmycin®, Polycyclidine® (Bristol Labs), Retet®, Rexamycin®, Robitet®, Sumycin®, Tetrachel (S)®, Tetracyn® (Pfizer), Tetrastatin®	5 µg, 30 µg	1.0 – 5.0
Ticarcillin	Ticar®	(ampicillin class)	
Tobramycin	Nebcin® (Eli Lilly)	10 µg	4.0 – 10.0
Triple Sulfa		Equal parts of: Sulfadiazine, Sulfamethazine, Sulfamerazine 300 µg	
Vancomycin	Vancocin® (Eli Lilly)	30 µg	25

[1]Not all drugs are available for disc antimicrobial susceptibility testing. The U.S. Food and Drug Administration has designated certain drugs as representative of their drug "class". Thus, for example, a penicillin G disc is used for testing for penicillin G, phenoxymethyl penicillin, and phenethicillin.

[2]The actual amount of anti-microbial agent in the disc may deviate from the labeled potency. The labeled amount of drug has to perform, within experimental error, as the labeled potency when present in a standardized disc when both are compared under standardized conditions as set forth by the U.S. Food and Drug Administration.

[3]The size of the zone of inhibition, depending upon its diameter, indicates resistance, sensitive, or intermediate. These designations may vary with the size of the zone of inhibition depending on the genus and species of organisms being examined. The package inserts of the manufacturers of the discs will usually indicate these relationships between the size of the zone of inhibition and the interpretation with regard to resistance.

[4]Serum levels indicated represent peak range of concentrations, but may vary with dose and time after dose that blood levels are measured.

[5]The ampicillin disc is used for testing for ampicillin and hetacillin susceptibility.

[6]Cephalothin discs are used for testing for cephalothin, cephaloridine, and cephalexin susceptibility.

[7]Clindamycin discs are used for testing for lincomycin and clindamycin susceptibility.

[8]Methicillin represents the penicillinase - resistant penicillin class: methicillin, oxacillin, nafcillin, cloxacillin, dicloxacillin.

[9]Oleandomycin represents the class: Oleandomycin, Trioleandomycin.

[10]Represents the penicillin class: penicillin G, phenoxymethyl penicillin, phenethicillin.

[11]Tetracycline represents the class: tetracycline, oxytetracycline, methacycline, doxycycline, demecloycline, minocycline, rolitetracycline, chlortetracycline.

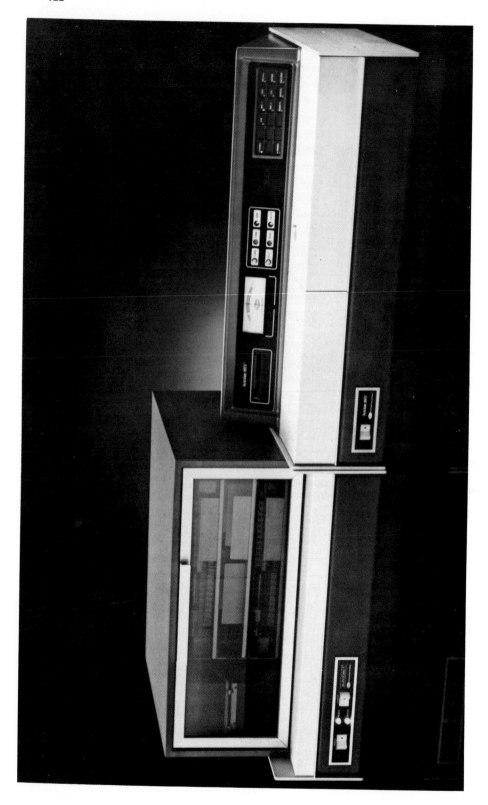

FIGURE 9. Light scattering device for determining MIC values. Autobac, Courtesy Pfizir Diagnostics Div., NYC, N.Y.

8. CASE HISTORIES

Understanding and education of the many ramifications of therapeutic drug monitoring, is best achieved (and perhaps by the only method) by analysis of day-to-day clinical situations, where unusual, bizarre, or other untoward pharmacologic and/or serum/plasma levels have been determined. It is intended that these brief case histories will provide the reader with examples of major, complex factors that must be considered when interpretating plasma drug levels and will tend to tie together much of the data and pertinent information presented throughout this text.

Source materials for these cases have been taken in part from personal experience, and also from a number of continuing education programs, workshops, seminars, informal meetings, as well as published accounts in the literature. For the reader's convenience the first section of cases deal with clinical ramifications, physiological, pharmacological, and pathological factors which can influence serum/plasma drug levels, while the second section addresses itself to analytical and methodological difficulties for blood drug level determinations.

CASE ONE

Phenytoin Pharmacokinetics

A 25 year old man with a two-year history of idiopathic epilepsy has a seizure at 9 p.m. without complications. Past history reveals that he had been on phenobarbital since the onset of the seizure disorder. One month ago phenobarbital was discontinued because seizure control was ineffective, and the patient was placed on phenytoin 100 mg p.o. b.i.d.

At 8 a.m. the morning after his seizure, the patient took phenytoin 100 mg p.o. He was seen by his physician at 11 a.m. when a serum phenytoin value of 11 mg/L was determined.

What are some of the pharmacological implications for this case including therapeutic range, steady-state phenytoin levels and dosage?

Discussion
1. In adults, the average therapeutic range for plasma phenytoin is 10 to 20 mg/L.
2. A steady state level is achieved 5 to 15 days after beginning oral therapy provided a loading dose is not used.
3. Absorption of phenytoin from the intestine is slow and variable. Peak blood concentrations are generally seen 4 to 24 hours after an oral dose. Since differences in bioavilibility occur with various phenytoin brands, plasma concentrations may reflect a change in preparation used.
4. If the concentration is the same or lower than 11 mg/L, it may suggest that an increase in the dosage schedule is indicated. It must be re-

membered that the half-life of the drug is stable with a constant dosage and when plasma concentrations are below 10 mg/L. With higher concentrations, an increase in dose will increase the half-life ("saturation kinetics"). For example, increasing the daily dose from 300 mg to 400 mg can double plasma concentration. The hydroxylated metabolites of phenytoin appear to saturate the metabolizing enzyme resulting in less phenytoin inactivation.

5. If the dose is increased, repeat the drug assay immediately before the sixth adjusted new dose.

Case Source   Dr. Mario Werner, Professor of Pathology (Laboratory of Medicine), The George Washington University Medical Center, Washington, D.C. Presented at ASCP Workshop - Clinical Consultation in Laboratory Medicine by Pathologists, ASCP Spring Meeting, April 1980, Atlanta, Ga., p. 5-7.

CASE TWO

Aminoglycoside Therapy

A patient R.K. with diabetes mellitus and hypertension develops septicemia with *Pseudomonas aeruginosa* after a urinary tract procedure. The patient is being started on gentamicin 80 mg I.V. every 12 hours and carbenicillin 5 gms I.V. every 6 hours. Because the patient has diseases that are associated with impairment of kidney function, the physician would like to make certain that the aminoglycoside dose is appropriate to optimize therapy and avoid or reduce toxicity.

Discussion

1. How many blood levels are necessary to get a reasonable estimate of the patients pharmacokinetic parameters?
   This can be accomplished with 2 blood levels, not necessarily a peak and a trough, from the same dosing interval. The time of the dose and the time of each blood level must be noted. *If the patient is stable,* blood levels may be obtained from 2 dosing intervals. Often, to be practical, a trough is drawn fromn dose A, just prior to dose B, then the peak obtained.
2. When should these blood levels be obtained?
   They may be obtained anytime in the dosing interval. They should not be obtained during the distribution phase. For the greatest amount of accuracy, the 2 levels should be separated by as much time as possible during that interval.
3. How often should this blood level information be obtained?
   If the patient has stable kidney function and an improving infectious disease picture, this information may not be needed at all. If the patients kidney function is dramatically and continually changing, or if the patient is deteriorating clinically, this information may be necessary every 24 - 72 hours.

4. Could this patient's carbenicillin therapy affect the aminoglycoside concentration determination?

It is well established that the *in vitro* mixing of aminoglycosides and pencillins, particularly carbenicillin and ticarcillin, results in decreased activity of the aminoglycoside. It is thought that this reaction is concentration dependent and may occur *in vivo*, particularly in patients with severly impaired kidney function.

5. Could this patient's carbenicillin therapy adversely affect the outcome of aminoglycoside therapy?

It is theoretically possible, and suspected, that carbenicillin or ticarcillin inactivation of aminoglycoside could contribute to adverse patient treatment. Presently, this is just a suspicion and its actual significance is in question.

6. What are the indications for obtaining serum drug concentrations in patients treated with aminoglycosides?
   1. Patients with dramatically changing renal function.
   2. Patients with acute renal failure.
   3. Patients with chronic renal failure whether or not they are receiving peritoneal-or hemo-dialysis.
   4. Patients in whom a lack of response is suspected to be due to inadequate drug therapy.
   5. Patients suspected of having drug toxicity.

Case Source   Dr. Thomas Cali, Assistant Professor, Clinical Pharmacy, University of Maryland School of Pharmacy, Presented at AACC Traveling TDM Program, May 8, 1980, Columbia, Maryland, pp. 42-44.

CASE THREE

Elevated Theophylline Levels

Your chemistry laboratory determines a serum theophylline level of 30 mg/L on patient T.C. On calling the medical resident he has no idea why the level is so high.

What information would help you evaluate this level?

Discussion

1. When was the level drawn in relation to the dose?

The level was drawn while T.C. was receiving an I.V. infusion.

2. What type of theophylline was being given and what was the dose?

Aminophylline at 0.9 mg/kg/hr.

3. How long had T.C. been receiving this dose?

3 days

4. How was the aminophylline started?

T.C. was given a loading dose of 6 mg/kg, then the infusion was started.

5. Was T.C. taking any medication prior to starting the aminophylline?

   The asthma patient had been controlled on 200 mg aminophylline every 6 hours for 6 months prior to this acute attack. The patient is taking no other medications.

6. Does the patient have any other diseases, e.g., congestive heart failure or liver disease?

   The patient is a long standing alcohol abuser with hepatic cirrhosis.

7. How would you evaluate this 30 mg/L serum level?

   The patient has at least two apparent reasons for this increased serum level. First T. C. had been taking his aminophylline religiously prior to his entering the emergency room. Therefore, he probably had a substantial amount of theophylline on board. Instead of giving the patient a loading dose of 6 mg/kg, the assumption that T. C. had a significant serum theophylline concentration should have been made and only a maintenance infusion started without the loading dose. Second, T. C. has a history of significant liver disease, which will probably decrease the speed at which theophylline is cleared from the body. Theophylline is metabolized primarily through the microsomal enzyme system which, in patients with hepatic cirrhosis, does not function as efficiently. There-fore, the maintenance infusion of 0.9 mg/kg of aminophylline in this patient is probably too much.

8. Recommendation?

   No loading dose should have been given and the maintenance infusion rate should have been 0.5 mg/kg/hr for the first 12 hours followed by 0.2 mg/kg/hr. This dosing should be followed with serum theophylline levels in at least 12 to 24 hours.

Case Source   Dr. Gordon Ireland, Assistant Professor of Clinical Phar-macy, University of Maryland School of Pharmacy and Clinical Pharmacist, VA Medical Center, Baltimore, Maryland. Presented at AACC Traveling TDM Program, May 1, 1980, Minneapolis, Minnesota, pp. 60-63.

CASE FOUR

Procainamide Kinetics

The rhythm strip of a 63 year old female patient receiving 500 mg of procainamide (PA) HCl every 4 hours for 7 days shows frequent PVCs 1 - 2 hours following dose. A sample of blood is drawn at the end of the dosing interval (4 hours after previous dose), and serum levels of PA and NAPA are 5 and 6 mg/l, respectively. The physician concludes that the patient is not responding to the drug, and that another drug is indicated because (1) the serum concentration of PA is in its therapeutic range, (2) the sum of PA and NAPA is in the therapeutic range, and (3) these serum levels are the lowest since the sample was drawn at the end of the dosing interval.

Discussion

Although reasons 1 and 2 are correct, reason 3 may not be. The physician is assuming that the drug is rapidly absorbed. If PA is slowly absorbed from the gut, peak serum concentrations can occur 2-4 hours after the dose is given. This case illustrates the potential pitfalls associated with drawing only one blood for PA and NAPA analysis.

Case Source   Dr. John Lima, Assistant Professor, Pharmacokinetics Laboratory, Division of Pharmacy Practice, College of Pharmacy, Ohio State University. Presented at AACC Traveling TDM Program, May 8, 1980, Columbia, Maryland, p. 76.

CASE FIVE

Procainamide Dosage Timing

A physician prescribes 500 mg of Procainamide hydrochloride (PA-HCl) every 3 hours for a 70 year old patient with a recent MI. He orders 3 blood samples drawn for PA analysis 1, 2, and 3 hours following the first dose of the drug. Results of this analysis show serum concentrations of PA of 1.7, 1.7, and 1.6 mg/l, respectively. The dose of PA·HCl is increased to 750 mg every 3 hours. A blood sample drawn 1 hour following this 750 mg dose contains a concentration of PA of 5.2 mg/l. Since the therapeutic range of PA is 4 - 10 mg/l, the physician is satisfied that 750 mg of PA·HCl every 3 hours will maintain serum concentrations of PA in its therapeutic range. Four days later the patient has minor signs of PA toxicity, and steady-state serum levels of PA and NAPA are 11 and 20 mg/l, respectively.

Discussion

The case illustrates the pitfalls associated with making conclusions regarding dose administration prior to achieving steady-state.

Case Source   Dr. John Lima, Assistant Professor, Pharmacokinetics Laboratory, Division of Pharmacy Practice, College of Pharmacy, Ohio State University. Presented at AACC Traveling TDM Program, May 8, 1980, Columbia, Maryland, pp. 76-77.

CASE SIX

Procainamide (PA) Serum Concentrations

A 176-lb. patient is receiving intravenously 4.0 gm of PA daily. His rhythm strip shows frequent PVCs. Steady-state serum concentrations of PA and NAPA are 2.78 and 3.1 mg/l, respectively.

Discussion

Although the dose of PA in this patient corresponds to that receommended in the literature, steady-state serum concentrations of PA are not in the therapeutic range. Based on these data, the daily dose of PA should be doubled. This case illustrates that the dose of PA cannot be relied upon to maintain serum concentrations of the drug and its metabolite in their respective therapeutic ranges.

Case Source   Dr. John Lima, Assistant Professor, Pharmacokinetics Laboratory, Division of Pharmacy Practice, College of Pharmacy, Ohio State University. Presented at AACC Traveling TDM Program, May 8, 1980, Columbia, Maryland, p. 77

CASE SEVEN

Aminoglycosides

Blood was received for B.T., a seriously ill patient, at 9:00 a.m. and the gentamicin level was reported to be 3.0 mg/L. The resident feels that the level is lower than expected. What may account for this result?

Discussion

1. When was the blood obtained in relation to the dose?
    Without knowing the answer to this question, the blood concentration would be meaningless. If this were a peak concentration, it may be too high. If this is neither a peak nor a trough, even knowing when the blood was drawn, it is much less useful than a peak or trough level.
2. What was the route of administration of the drug in relation to the time the level was obtained?
    With intramuscularly administered gentamicin, consideration must be given to the absorptive phase (30 to 90 minutes). If the blood was obtained significantly outside of this time interval, the relationship of the level (3.0 mg/L) to the actual peak concentration cannot be determined.
3. What patient characteristics would tend to interfere with the interpretation of the level?
    Increased serum concentrations of aminoglycosides have been noted in patients who are febrile as well as in patients with a low hematocrit.
4. How was the sample handled?
    Depending upon various factors, the aminoglycoside concentration may decline when standing at room temperature for prolonged periods of time. Hemolysis may increase the drug concentration by liberating the drug from the red blood cell, or it may affect the sensitivity of some assay procedures.

5. What concommitant drug therapy might interfere with the drug concentration?

Fortunately, aminoglycoside concentrations are not affected by many drugs. High concentrations of heparin may affect the serum concentration, as well as heparin in a vacutainer, or drawing the sample through a venous access site containing heparin.

6. What is the accuracy of testing procedure used?

For every test result, the accuracy of the testing procedure needs to be established.

7. When should the trough level be drawn?

The trough level is the lowest drug concentration seen during a dosing interval. This occurs just prior to the next dose of drug. The trough level is drawn immediately before the next dose-whether the drug is administered intravenously or intramuscularly.

8. When should the peak level be drawn?

The peak concentration is the highest concentration of drug during a dosing interval *after* the distribution phase is complete.

Case Source   Dr. Mario Werner, Professor of Pathology (Laboratory Medicine), The George Washington University Medical Center, Washington, D. C. Presented as ASCP Workshop — Clinical Consultation in Laboratory Medicine by Pathologists, ASCP Spring Meeting, April 1980, Atlanta, Ga., pp. 39-41.

CASE EIGHT

Low Theophylline Blood Levels

A 54 year old while male presented to the emergency room with acute exacerbation of his asthma. He had been taking 200 mg aminophylline every 6 hours. A blood level drawn was 5.0 mg/L which is lower than the medical resident expected. What may accont for this result?

Discussion

1. Non-compliance to medication.

This is the primary reason for therapeutic failure in any course of therapy.

2. When was the blood obtained in relation to the dose?

If the level was drawn 6 hours after the dose it would constitute a trough level at the lower boundary of the therapeutic range. In spite of this, the level is not sufficient in this patient so the dose should be increased to achieve a higher trough level, e.g., 8-10 mg/L.

If this level was drawn 2 hours after the last dose it would coincide with the peak serum concentration of the oral drug. This concentration is sub-therapeutic for a peak level and the dose should be increased.

3. What was the route of administration in relation to the time the level was obtained?

Intravenous dosing would cause a peak serum about 0-½ hr after the dose was administered.

Intramuscular administration, although painful (possibly because of the alkaline preparation), is rapidly absorbed and achieves a peak serum level similar to I.V. dosing.

Oral dosing is also completely (90-95%) absorbed with a peak level occurring 1-2 hrs after the dose on an empty stomach and later if taken with food.

Sustained release products would cause a more even blood level with later and lower peaks and higher troughs although the total amount of drug absorbed might be the same as other oral forms.

Rectal suppositories are erratically and unreliably absorbed.

4. Patient characteristics which might change levels.

This lower level may be due to the fact that this patient is a heavy smoker. Smokers tend to clear the drug from their bodies faster than non-smokers secondary to the induction of drug-metabolizing enzymes in the liver by compounds contained in cigarette smoke or their metabolites.

Other factors which may increase blood levels include liver disease and ngestive heart failure because of decreased clearance of the drug.

5. Concommitant drug therapy.

Concurrent administration of theophylline and phenobarbital may cause an increase in the hepatic clearance of the theophylline and therefore lower the blood levels. This increased clearance is caused by phenobarbital stimulation of microsomal enzymes production in the liver which then increases the rate of theophylline metabolism.

Case Source   Dr. Gordon Ireland, Assistant Professor of Clinical Pharmacy, Universitty of Maryland School of Pharmacy and Clinical Pharmacist, VA Medical Center, Baltimore, Maryland. Presented at AACC Traveling TDM Program, May 1, 1980, Minneapolis, Minnesota, pp. 55-60.

CASE NINE

Acetaminophen Overdose

In February, 1978, a 19-year-old woman was transferred to St. Anthony Hospital Poisoning Treatment Center, 24 hr after admission to a local community hospital because she had ingested an overdose of acetaminophen. The patient's family physician indicated that 6 hr before her admission to the community hospital, the patient had ingested 75 0.5-g tablets of a proprietary medication subsequently identified as acetaminophen.

Laboratory data at the time of admission revealed an erythrocyte count of 4.6 million/mm^3, a hemoglobin concentration of 145 gm/L, a hemotocrit of 40%, and a leukocyte count of 10,600 cells/mm^3, with a normal differential count. Platelets were considered to be adequate in number. Serum electrolytes were: 142 MMO1/L; potassium, 4.8 MMO1/L; chloride 101 MMO1/L, and CO_2, 30 MMO1/L. Other clinical chemical values were: calcium 96 mg/L; phosphorous was 45 mg/L, alkaline phosphatase, 25 U/L aspartate aminotransferase, 850 U/L; alanine aminotransferase, 2050 U/L; and bilirubin 23 mg/L. The blood glucose concentration was 1.05 g/L.

The patient was admitted to the Intensive Care Unit. A sample of blood was submitted to the toxicology reference laboratory for emergency determination of serum acetaminophen concentration. The acetaminophen concentrations at the time of admission to community hospital was found to be 400 mg/L.

About 6 hr after the initial determination of acetaminophen concentration and biochemical profile at this hospital, the patient was noted to be confused and to have developed scleral icterus. No asterixis was noted and no bleeding developed. A repeat determination of acetaminophen revealed that the acetaminophen concentration was now 370 mg/L. This persistently high acetaminophen concentration, combined with neurological and hepatic deterioration, suggested severe acetaminophen poisoning. The aspartate aminotransferase concentration was now 40 K U/L, the alanine aminotransferase 720 K U/L, and the bilirubin 30 mg/L. The prothrombin time was normal, as was the blood ammonia concentration.

The patient was transferred to the Center for further therapy, and was given 140 mg of acetylcysteine per kilogram body weight by mouth, plus a maintenance dose of 70 mg/kg orally administered, shortly after her arrival at the Center. A standing dose of 70 mg/kg was given every 4 hr for the next 3 days, for a total of 17 such maintenance doses. During this time, the patient was carefully evaluated for change in neurological status, bleeding, respiratory complications, fluid and electrolyte imbalance, and other problems. Her hepatic status was followed very closely.

Twelve hours after she was admitted to St. Anthony Hospital, her neurological status had deteriorated significantly, and she had asterixis and evidence of hepatic coma. She was moderately jaundiced and the liver was enlarged and tender. The SGOT value exceeded 100 K U/L. The serum alkaline phosphatase activity was 5.50 K U/L, 857 of which appeared to be liver-derived. The leukocyte count was 17,500 cells/mm³, and the serum acetaminophen concentration was 85 mg/L.

The patient began to improve clinically 24 hr after admission to St. Anthony Hospital. The SGOT was noted to be 30 K U/L and the SGPT 250 K U/L. The bilirubin was 26 mg/L. By this time the patient's neurological status was significantly improved. Her asterixis and confusion had disappeared, and the acetaminophen value was 20 mg/L.

She continued to improve, and was discharged from the hospital on the 10th day after this admission, at which time results were normal.

About a month later her liver was biopsied, and no significant abnormalitites were seen. She was considered to be well.

Discussion

1. What are the side-effects of acetaminophen dosage?

   Side effects of treatment with acetaminophen are negligible in ordinary therapeutic dosage. The drug is well tolerated, does not cause gastrointestinal bleeding, and is not believed to affect platelet function.

Hepatic disease as a result of normal doses is almost unknown. Some dizziness, nausea, and mild psychic effects have been described.

The principal problem with acetaminophen is the severe liver disorder caused by massive overdoses, a problem first described about 10 years ago, in Britain. At first, it was believed to be a phenomenon confined to a relatively limited genetic population in the British Isles, but more recently it has been reported in almost every country wherein the drug is used. Clearly, the problem arises from a rate-limited shift from the usual metabolism of acetaminophen.

In the presence of massive overdoses of the drug, the liver's ability to provide sulfhydryl groups for the formation of its sulfate metabolite is overwhelmed, and a disproportionate amount of the hepatotoxic osymetabolites, cysteinate, and mercaptate are produced. The production of these more toxic metabolites increases with the dose, and this may totally destroy the liver. If the disorder is recognized, a large excess of sulfhydryl groups can be provided by administering a sulfhydryl donor such as acetylcysteine. This apparently helps protect the liver. Other sulfhydryl donors such as glutathione and D-penicillamine have been utilized successfully, but are much more difficult to give.

2. How should specimens be obtained?

Specimens should be obtained on admission to hospital if at least 4 hr have passed since the overdose of acetaminophen was taken. A second specimen should be obtained 4 hr after that and the half-life determined; if it exceeds 4 hr and the total concentration exceeds 150 g/L, there is a very high probability that liver disorder will be detected.

3. What is the metabolic fate of acetaminophen?

The metabolic disposition of acetaminophen is interesting. The excretion of the drug varies with the dose ingested. In ordinary therapeutic doses, about 4.2% is excreted as acetaminophen, unchanged. Two primary metabolites are noted, the glucuronide and the sulfate, and in addition a small percentage of the ingested dose may be excreted as the mercaptate and the cysteinate, both of which are the result of oxidative metabolism of acetaminophen. An intermediate oxymetabolite, which has not been identified, is believed to be the toxic material associated with liver necrosis. It has been demonstrated that this oxymetabolite can bind covalently to liver macromolecules and cause destruction of the hepatocyte function. Fortunately, the oxymetabolite is a very minor product in acetaminophen metabolism under ordinary circumstances. The liver can readily provide glutathione for the formation of the sulfate metabolite, but if the ingested dose exceeds 2 g, the oxymetabolite may increase in concentration, with a relative decrease in the proportion excreted as sulfates and an increase in the excretion of the cysteinate and mercaptate conjugates of acetaminophen. After a single dose of 30 g, one that is almost always associated with severe liver disorder, the percentages of the excreted drug may appear as follows: acetaminophen, 13.8%, acetaminophen glucuronide, 32.7%, acetaminophen sulfate, 8.66%, and acetaminophen cysteinate and mercaptate, 44.8%.

4. What is the clinical protocol for management of acetaminophen overdoses?

When a patient is admitted who has ingested more than one or two tablets (if a small child) or more than five or 10 tablets (if an adult), acetaminophen should be measured within 4 hr of the ingestion, and if the results exceed 150 mg/L there is a significant probability of acute hepatic disorder. If the initially determined value is less than this 4 hr after ingestion, the probability of hepatic necrosis is extremely small. If the patient is hospitalized and therapy with acetylcysteine begun for acetaminophen intoxication, the laboratory should be prepared to repeat the acetaminophen determination approximately 4 hr after the initial determination. A demonstrated half-life of longer than 4 hr would be consistent with a very high probability of acetaminophen-induced liver toxicity. All patients should have emergency baseline studies of hepatic function on admission, including SGOT, SGPT, and glutamyltransferase. These should be repeated daily until all evidence of liver disorder has passed.

The now recommended protocol for management calls for the administration of a loading dose of acetylcysteine of 140 mg/kg, and a maintenance dose of 70 mg of acetylcysteine per kilogram body weight every 4 hr for 3 days. Throughout this period and for about three to four days afterwards, or until the results of liver-function tests return to normal, SGOT, SGPT, GGTP should be measured.

Acetaminophen should be monitored at eight-hour intervals until concentrations reach 50 mg/L or less. In patients with severe hepatic necrosis this may take several days. If adequate glutathione is provided through the administration of acetylcysteine, one may expect to see a reasonably good disposition of the overdose of acetaminophen.

Case Source   Dr. Daniel T. Teitelbaum, President, Center for Toxicology, Man and Environment, Inc., Denver, Colorado. Presented in AACC Therapeutic Drug Monitoring Continuing Education and Quality Control Program, Nov. 1979, pp. 1-5.

CASE TEN

Valproic Acid

In this case, valproic acid was used in treating a 26-year-old woman(B.V.) suffering from post-anoxic myoclonus. Action myoclonus has frequently been described as a complication of cerebral hypoxia.

The patient had a long-standing history of steroid-dependent asthma. She suffered a respiratory arrest and, when found, was unconscious. The duration of the hypoxic episode is unknown.

Admitted to the intensive-care unit, she was maintained on artificial ventilation for six days. When she regained consciousness she was severly incapacitated by myoclonus. Several anticonvulsants were tried (phenobarbital, phenytoin, nitrazepam, and diazepam) but were ineffective. Clonazepam produced mild improvement. The patient was discharged with instructions to take 10 mg of clonazepam twice daily.

Several months later, she was readmitted because of violent jerking movements, which appeared when she tried to stand. She could not walk, and suffered from rapid, labored respirations, tachycardia, and eventual exhaustion.

All laboratory investigations, including a complete blood count, urinalysis, liver-function tests, and serum urea nitrogen and serum glucose value, were normal. Results of the one electroencephalogram were normal.

The patient was profoundly hypotonic. Knee jerks were pendular, the plantar responses were flexor, and sensation was normal. Her ability to perform rapid alternating movements was impaired.

Treatment of the patient with valproic acid was begun at an initial dosage of 200 mg four times daily (15 mg/kg per day), a dosage that was slowly increased to 650 mg four times daily (50 mg/kg per day), where-upon the myoclonus decreased and the patient found she could walk unaided. Serum valproic acid concentrations at this dosage varied from 110 to 145 mg/L. After she had received this dosage of valporate for two weeks, the patient's serum aspartate amino transferase and alanine aminotransferase activities were 185 and 132 U/L, respectively (normal: < 40 U/L for each).

The dosage of valproic acid was reduced to 450 mg four times daily (35 mg/kg per day), and the patient remained free of myoclonus. Administration of clonazepam, 20 mg/day, was continued. Serum valproic acid ranged from 72 to 103 mg/L. Six weeks after initiating this lower dosage, the transferase values returned to normal and the patient was still free of myoclonus. Eight weeks after the start of the present regimen and 20 weeks after starting valporate therapy, a blood-sample was drawn for measurement of valproate.

Discussion

Post-anoxic action myoclonus, sometimes called the Lance-Adams syndrome, can result in severe and prolonged disability. Several reports have shown that anticonvulsants such as phenobarbital, phenytoin, diazepam, nitrazepam, and carbamazepine are largely ineffective in controlling the severe myoclonus that occurs when these patients attempt to stand or walk, or which can be elicited by anxiety or other stimuli.

It is believed that some cases of Lance-Adams syndrome may be due to localized depletion of gamma-aminobutyrate and that the effectiveness of valproate is related to its ability to increase it.

The patient described here began to improve and eventually was able to care for herself. She had suffered only negligible intellectual decline.

Case Source   Dr. Roger L. Boeckx, Assistant Director of Clinical Chemistry, Children's Hospital, National Medical Center, Washington, D.C. Presented in AACC Therapeutic Drug Monitoring Continuing Education and Quality Control Program. Dec. 1979. p.

CASE ELEVEN

Valproic Acid in Klippel-Trenauny-Weber Syndrome

This is a case of the Klippel-Trenauny-Weber syndrome complicated by a severe seizure disorder attributed to progressively worsening asymmetric hydrocephalus. The case is unusual in that it describes the use of valproic acid to treat severe seizure disorder in an infant.

E.L., a four-month-old girl, was transferred from another hospital for the continued treatment of sepsis and a severe seizure disorder, and for evaluation of multiple congenital anomalies.

She had been hospitalized four times since birth for treatment of severe pneumonia. Her most recent admission to the referring hospital was because of fever, lethargy, and respiratory distress. A severe and progressive asymetric hydrocephalus, possible sepsis, and worsening seizure disorder prompted her transfer. Repeated bouts of infection prompted cancellation of shunt therapy for the hydrocephalus.

On admission, the patient was receiving 200 mg of ampicillin each 6 h, 50 mg of gentamicin every 2 h, 70 mg of primidone twice a day, and 40 mg of carbamazepine twice a day.

The hematocrit was 35.7%; the leukocyte count was 9700/μL with 38% neutrophils and 1% band forms. The platelet concentration was normal. The serum sodium concentration was 141 mmol/L, the potassium 3.3 mmol/L, the chloride 96 mmol/L, and the carbon dioxide content 27 mmol/L. Results of urinalysis were normal. Phenobarbital and carbamazepine concentrations were 32 and 2 mg/L, respectively. Increasing her carbamazepine dosage to 50 mg twice a day increased the concentration in serum to 5 mg/L, but had little effect on the frequency of seizures.

Valproic acid was added to her regimen in an attempt to better control the seizures. The patient was started at a dosage of 25 mg each 6 hr (22 mg/kg per day). A peak value after three days of therapy was 35 mg/L. The dosage was increased to 35 mg each 6 hr (30 mg/kg per day), resulting in a concentration of 56 mg/L in the serum but with little clinical improvement. A week later, at a dosage of 40 mg every 6 hours (36 mg/kg/day) the peak serum valproate values increased to 75 mg/L. However, phenobarbital values increased to 43 mg/L. The patient still had frequent seizures.

The dosage of valproic acid was further increased to 50 mg every 6 hr (44 mg/kg per day), and the primidone dosage was decreased to 60 mg twice a day. Seizures substantially decreased, but there were still occasional episodes of seizure activity. Serum drug concentrations on this regimen were: phenobarbital, 22 mg/L; carbamazepine, 3 mg/L; valproate, 102 mg/L. At present, the patients anticonvulsant regimen is: primidone, 60 mg twice daily; carbamazepine, 50 mg twice daily; and valproate, 50 mg four times a day. There are fewer seizures. One week after starting this dosage regimen, a blood-sample was drawn for measurement of anticonvulsants.

Discussion

Klippel-Trenaunay-Weber syndrome, a rare condition, usually consists of unilaterally located nevi, varicose veins, and hypertrophy of soft tissues and bone. This case is a severe manifestation in an infant in whom severe central nervous system damage, with hydrocephalus and unremitting seizures, is an additional complication. Treatment with primidone and carbamazepine in therapeutic dosage and with documented therapeutic concentrations in the serum resulted in little resolution of the seizure disorder. Valproic acid was added and was only moderately beneficial at first. The initial dosage of 22 mg/kg per day did not result in therapeutic concentrations; an increased dosage (44 mg/kg per day) eventually resulting in clinical improvement, with concentrations in serum exceeding 100 mg/L.

Despite the improvement in the seizure disorder, the prognosis for this severly damaged child is very poor.

Case Source Dr. Roger L. Boeckx, Assistant Director of Clinical Chemistry, Children's Hospital, National Medical Center, Washington, D.C. Presented in AACC Therapeutic Drug Monitoring Continuing Education and Quality Control Program, Dec. 1979, pp. 1-2.

CASE TWELVE

Phenytoin Non-Compliance

T.G., a 27-year-old unemployed white man, was brought to the hospital emergency department by ambulance in a semi-conscious state. His wife, who accompanied him and who had called the ambulance, reported that he had been under treatment for epilepsy since childhood, but had been seizure-free for almost two years. For the past month the patient had been severely depressed because of his inability to find work, and had been irregular in his sleeping and eating habits. In addition, he had sometimes neglected to take his prescribed phenytoin, and on the morning in question he had a typical grand mal seizure.

Immediate management consisted only of observation and monitoring of vital signs. After about 4 hr he awoke from his deep sleep and, except for mild confusion with respect to time and place, appeared to be perfectly normal.

Additional history obtained at that time revealed that the patient had for the past three weeks taken less than one-quarter of his prescribed daily dose of 400 mg of phenytoin. He justified this action to himself on the basis of his long freedom from seizures, which led him to believe he no longer needed the medication. Moreover, he related his inability to find work to his continuing dependence on phenytoin, and he hoped that stopping the drug would in some way help him to find a job.

A plasma phenytoin assay showed a concentration of 3.5 mg/L. The patient was then given a single oral loading dose of phenytoin of 700 mg, and urged to recommence his regular daily maintenance dose of 200 mg twice daily.

Seen one week later in clinic, he reported that he felt well and had not had another seizure. The plasma phenytoin concentration was now 14.7 mg/L, so he was advised to carry on with his established drug regimen. In addition, arrangements were made for a return to the clinic in six months for repeat of the plasma phenytoin measurement, and reassessment.

Discussion

This case illustrates the commonest single problem in long term phenytoin therapy-non compliance-and indicates how monitoring phenytoin in plasma may be of value in dealing with the problem.

As with any other disease that requires long-term medication, patient compliance is a major factor in the success or failure of drug therapy in epilepsy. In the case of phenytoin, it has been estimated that 30-40% of plasma values of < 10 mg/L are the result of the patient failing to take (or receive) his prescribed medication. This may be done inadvertently, through misunderstanding or carelessness, or deliberately, in an attempt to deny the need, or for various other reasons. In any case, the situation is further complicated by the unpredictability of seizures, so that there may be long non-compliance before the consequences become apparent.

In a patient with a history of non-compliance, it has been shown that regular clinic visits, with measurement of plasma phenytoin at each visit, serve as an effective stimulus to improve compliance. In addition, such visits provide a valuable opportunity to help the patient understand his condition, as well as objective data on which to base logical decisions about modifying drug dosage.

Case Source Dr. J. Gilbert Hill, Head of Service Division, Department of Biochemistry, Hospital for Sick Children, Toronto, Ontario. Presented in AACC Therpeutic Drug Monitoring Continuing Education and Quality Control Program, Feb. 1980, p. 1.

CASE THIRTEEN

Theophylline Dosage with Liver Cirrhosis

A 60 year old man with a history of Laennec's cirrhosis documented by biopsy was admitted to a hospital because of severe congestive heart failure and bronchospasm. Continuous intravenous theophylline therapy was instituted with an intravenous loading dose of 5.6 mg/kg/20 minutes followed by a maintenance dose of 0.9 mg/dg/hour. After one hour of therapy, a theophylline assay in blood produced a value of 15 mg/L.

Discussion

1. Theophylline is a 1,3-dimethyl xanthine which acts by inhibiting the enzyme phosphodiesterase, thereby increasing cyclic AMP and decreasing the formation of 5'AMP. One of the drug's primary effects is to relax the bronchial smooth muscles especially if the bronchioles are constricted as in asthma and congestive heart failure. This results in an increase in vital capacity. Theophylline also increases cardiac output, stimulates respiration and enhances diuresis. The therapeutic range of theophylline is 8 to 20 mg/L. It has been suggested that the target serum concentration should be about 10 mg/L within one hour after the loading dose and in case of continuous infusion. The drug is partially demethylated and oxidized in the liver with a plasma half-life of about 4 hours. The half-life is prolonged in liver disease.

2. Recommended dosage and therapeutic blood concentration are for a young patient with asthma who shows no evidence of congestive heart failure or hepatic disease. Since 90% of theophylline is biotransformed in the liver, it can be anticipated that halving of the maintenance dose to 0.45 mg/kg/hour is appropriate in the present case. Both the severe congestive heart and the cirrhosis contribute to a reduction of hepatic blood perfusion. Possible signs that a further decrease in dosage may be indicated are diarrhea, hypotension or arrhythmias. A repeat theophylline assay 24 hours after initiation of therapy is indicated.

Case Source Dr. Mario Werner, Professor of Pathology (Laboratory Medicine), The George Washington University Medical Center, Washington, D.C. Presented at ASCP Workshop - Clinical Consultation in Laboratory Medicine by Pathologists, ASCP Spring Meeting, April 1980, Atlanta, Ga., pp. 13-14.

CASE FOURTEEN

Quinidine Therapy and Purpura

A 55 year old woman with a history of atrial fibrillation had been effectively controlled on quinidine 200 mg. p.o., q.i.d. for one month. She was seen by her physician because of the abrupt onset of numerous purpuric lesions located on her extremities and trunk as well as hemorrhagic oral vesicles. Physical exam was otherwise unremarkable. Hematogram was normal except for a platelet count of 25,000/μl. Prothrombin time and activated partial thromboplastin time were within normal limits. A blood specimen was obtained two hours after her last dose and was analyzed fluorometrically for quinidine. The laboratory reported a value of 4 mg/L.

Discussion

1. The therapeutic range for plasma quinidine assayed fluorometrically is 3 to 6 μg/ml. Therapeutic responses are uncommon below a value of 3 mg/l, while toxicity is usually seen with levels in excess of 10 mg/L. The maximal absorption occurs 1 to 3 hours after and may persist for 8 hours. The biologic half-life is 5 hours.
2. Since there is no evidence of an ongoing infectious process or a coagulation factor deficiency, thrombocytopenic purpura secondary to quinidine therapy definitely should be considered. This is a rare but serious complication of quinidine therapy. The immune-mediated phenomenon occurs primarily in female patients over 50 years old. Quinidine may attach directly to the platelet surface thus forming a haptenic complex that elicits antibody formation. When antibody complexes with the drug already attached to the platelet, complement activation and platelet lysis occur. Alternatively, the drug-antibody complex may form in the circulation prior to attaching itself to the platelet. The severity of the thrombocytopenia does not appear to be dose related.
3. Quinidine should be discontinued. This will often terminate the bleeding even while the platelet count is still low. The platelet count usually returns to normal within 3 to 14 days.

Case Source Dr. Mario Werner, Professor of Pathology (Laboratory Medicine), The George Washington University Medical Center, Washington, D.C. Presented at ASCP Workshop - Clinical Consultation in Laboratory Medicine by Pathologists, ASCP Spring Meeting, April 1980, Atlanta, Ga., pp. 16-17.

CASE FIFTEEN

Digoxin Intoxication

A 65 year old widow with a history of congestive heart failure had been maintained on digoxin 0.25 mg p.o.q.d. and furosemide 40 mg p.o.q.d. for several months. She was encouraged to drink citrus juices to supplement her potassium intake. The following laboratory values were obtained three hours after oral dose:

	Plasma Digoxin ng/ml	Serum K+ meq/l	Serum Creatinine mg/dl
January	1.6	3.5	1.0
February	1.4	3.4	0.9
March	1.8	3.1	1.1

When the patient visited her physician in March, she complained of nausea, irregular heart rhythm and seeing yellow lights.

Discussion

1. An acceptable therapeutic range for plasma digoxin determined by radioimmunoassay is 0.6 to 1.6 ng/ml with values greater than 2.4 ng/ml being considered toxic. About 75% of the drug is absorbed after an oral dose with a peak blood concentration seen 1 to 5 hours. The plasma half-life is 36 hours.

2. The primary effect of digoxin is its ability to increase the force of myocardial contraction. However, digoxin toxicity results in inhibition of the sodium/potassium activated adenine triphosphatase which is responsible for the active transport of sodium and potassium across the cardiac cell membrane. This results in a decrease in intracellular potassium and an increase in intracellular sodium which allows for the occurrence of extrasystoles. Therefore, especially when a kaljuretic drug such as furosemide is administered, supplemental potassium is needed. In this particular patient, the dietary potassium intake was probably inadequate, and supplemental KC1 should be prescribed.

   Since digoxin is eliminated in the urine by glomerular filteration, an elevated serum creatinine would suggest lowering of the maintenance dose of digoxin. This is not a consideration in the patient.

3. The combination of a slightly elevated plasma digoxin level with hypokalemia probably explains the patient's symptomatology of digoxin toxicity.

4. It is recommended that the patient's digoxin and furosemide be withheld for a day and supplemental potassium be administered, thus attempting to normalize the digoxin and potassium level. Repeat the digoxin and potassium assays after 24 hours. An electrocardiogram may be helpful now and possibly again in 24 hours.

Case Source   Dr. Mario Werner, Professor of Pathology (Laboratory Medicine), The George Washington University Medical Center, Washington, D.C. Presented at ASCP Workshop - Clinical Consultation in Laboratory Medicine by Pathologists, ASCP Spring Meeting, April 1980, Atlanta, Ga., pp. 19-21.

CASE SIXTEEN

HPLC Interference in Procainamide/NAPA Assay

A serum specimen was referred to the therapeutic drug monitoring laboratory (no clinical history provided) with a request for a procainamide/NAPA serum concentration. Upon HPLC analysis, the following data was obtained:

> Procainamide - 82.3 mg/liter
> NAPA - 4.8 mg/liter

The laboratory supervisor was notified of the grossly elevated procainamide value, and a conforming assay was indicated. The repeat assay obtained identical values. What are the practical implications of these determinations?

Discussion

1. The case illustrates the requirements for two important pieces of data that need accompany each request for a drug assay in the therapeutic drug monitoring laboratory:

   (a) *Complete* medication history of the patient.
   (b) Extensive interference studies data need be established and maintained on file for each given system of analysis.

2. The level of procainamide obtained in this specimen is absurd, even in fatal overdose cases, and should immediately alert the laboratory to analytical error or drug (or other endogenous substance) interference with the given method of analysis. Since the quality control data and repeat assay value show excellent correlation and results, an analytical interference was suspected.

3. A detailed medication history obtained from the hospital (after the fact) revealed the following drug regimen: digoxin, quinidine, propoxphene and Colace® (dioctyl sodium sulfosuccinate). It was interesting to note that no procainamide was indicated to have been administered, yet the analytical data suggested its presence.

Drug interference data revealed none of the above administered medications would interfere with this method of analysis, with the exception of Coloce® which has not been previously screened. Analytical data revealed that Colace® exhibited similar chromatographic characteristics when taken through the system of analysis, as that of procainamide. This would suggest a solution to the grossly elevated "procainamide" chromatographic peak, but would not explain the presence of the active metabolite, NAPA.

4. A detailed consultation with the clinical pathologist revealed that this patient indeed had been administered procainamide, but on a STAT basis, and such data had not been entered on the medication record. Analysis of the serum specimen by an alternative method (EMIT®), revealed the presence of 6.8 mg/liter procainamide, which had been "masked" in the interfering peak in the HPLC system. This data was then released to the submitted hospital.

Case Source George Morrell, Technical Director, MDS Health Group, Inc., Holmdel, New Jersey, and Dr. Irwin J. Hollander, Department of Pathology, Grand View Hospital, Sellersville, Pennsylvanna, Unpublished Patient Data, April 1980.

Appendix

GLOSSARY OF TERMS IN THERAPEUTIC DRUG MONITORING

Absorption: Process of uptake of one drug and/or metabolite from one site of administration into the systemic circulation.

Action vs. Effect: The effect of a drug is an alternation of function of the structure or process upon which the drug acts. It is common to use the term action as a synonym for effect. However, action precedes effect. Action is the alternation or condition that brings about the desired effect.

Active Transport: The energy-dependent movement of a substance through a biological membrane against an electrochemical gradient. It is characterized as follows:

- (a) The drug is transported from a region of lower to one of higher electrochemical activity;
- (b) Metabolic poisons interfere with transport.
- (c) The transport rate approaches an asymptote (i.e., saturates) as concentration increases;
- (d) The transport system usually shows a requirement for specific chemical structures;
- (e) Closely related chemicals are competitive for the transport system.

Many drugs are secreted from the renal tubules or into the bile by active transport, but the role of active transport of drugs in the distribution into the body compartments and tissues is less well known.

Area Under the Curve: The integral of drug blood level over time from zero to infinity. This is a measure of quantity of drug absorbed in the body.

Bioavailability: The relative amount of drug from an administered dosage form which enters the systemic circulation and the resulting rate at which the drug appears in the bloodstream.

Biological Half-Life: The time in hours necessary to reduce the drug concentration in the blood, plasma or serum to one-half after equilibrium is reached. The biological half-life is influenced by various factors including dosage, variation in urinary excretion and urinary pH, inter-patient variation, age, protein binding, disease states (especially renal and liver dysfunction), and interactions of other drugs.

The equation of Van Rossum and Tomey demonstrates the pharmacokinetic relationship between the biologic half-life ($t_{1/2}$) after a single dose and the steady-state blood concentration of that drug:

$$C = 1.44 \left[\frac{(Q)}{(\Delta t)} \frac{(t_{1/2})}{\frac{(Dose_a)}{(Ct_0)}} \right]$$

Where, Q: Maintenance dose

$Dose_a$: Amount of drug administered

Ct_0: "Zero" time plasma concentration of the drug

Δt: Dosage internal

Loss of drug from the body as described by one biologic half-life, means the elimination of the administered parent drug (including metabolite(s)) by urinary excretion, metabolism or other elimination route.

Biopharmaceutics: The physical and chemical properties of the drug, the dosage form, and the biological effectiveness of a drug (i.e., drug availability).

Biophase: The molecular level of the drug-receptor site of action in the body.

Biotransformation: Most drugs are acted upon by enzymes in the body and converted to metabolic derivatives called metabolites. The process of conversion is called biotransformation. Metabolites are usually more polar and less lipid-soluble than the parent drug because of the introduction of oxygen into the molecule, hydrolyzed to yield more highly polar groups, or conjugation with a highly polar substance.

Blood, Plasma or Serum Levels: The concentration in blood, plasma and serum (or other biological fluids, e.g., saliva) after administration of a given dosage by a particular route of administration. Blood, plasma, or serum level curves are plots of drug concentrations versus time on numeric or semi-log graph paper.

Brand Name or Drug Specimen: A drug product, labeled with a registered trademark of a particular company.

Compartment: An entry which can be described by a definite volume and a concentration of drug contained in that volume. Experimental data can then be explained by fitting into various 'compartment' models.

Dosage Form: The pharmaceutical form containing the active drug(s) and vehicle substances necessary in formulating a medicament of desired dosage, volume, and application form.

Dosage Regimen: The systemized dosage schedule for therapy, i.e., the time intervals at which a certain dose size must be administered in order to produce clinical effectiveness or to maintain therapeutic concentration in the body.

Dose: Amount of drug to be administered.

Drug-Receptor Interaction: The combination of a drug molecule with the receptor for which it has affinity, and the initiation of a pharmacologic response by its intrinsic activity.

Drug Resistance: The decrease in responsiveness of micro-organisms, neoplasms, or pests to chemotherapeutic agents, antineoplastics or pesticides. It is the survival of normally unresponsive cells which then pass the genetic factors of resistance on to their progeny.

Efficacy: Efficacy denotes the property of the drug to achieve the desired response. Efficacy is one of the primary determinations of the choice of a drug.

Excretion: The final elimination of drug(s) from the body's systemic circulation via the kidney into the urine, via bile into the intestines and saliva into feces, via sweat, skin, or milk.

Facilitated Diffusion: When a drug substance moves more rapidly through a biological membrane than can be accounted for by the process of simple diffusion. It is believed to be due to the presence of a special molecule, called a carrier, within the membrane, with which carrier the transported substance combines. It differs from active transport in that facilitated diffusion will only transport a molecule along its electrochemical gradient.

Generic Name: A drug product marketed under the nonproprietary or chemical (common) name of that particular substance.

Initial Dose (or Loading Dose): A dose size used in initiating therapy so as to yield therapeutic concentration(s) which will result in clinical effectiveness.

Ionic Diffusion: If a drug is ionized, the transport properties are modified. The probability of penetrating the membrane is a function of the potential difference or electrical gradient across the membrane, and of concentration. A cationic drug molecule will be repelled from the previous charge on the outside of the membrane, and only those molecules with a high kinetic energy will pass through the ion barrier.

LADME System: The complex dynamic process of liberation of an active ingredient from the dosage form, its absorption into systemic circulation, its distribution and metabolism and the excretion of the drug from the body.

Maintenance Dose: The dose size required to maintain the clinical effectiveness or therapeutic concentration for a given dosage regimen.

Membranes: The physical barrier to transport of drugs in the body. It is lipoidal in nature and consists of a double row of phospholipids sandwiched between one layer of protein.

Metabolism: The sum of all the clinical reactions for biotransformation of endogenous and exogenous substances which take place in the living cell.

Non-ionic Diffusion and Passive Transport: Molecules in solution move in a purely random fashion, providing they are not charged and moving in an electrical gradient. Such random movement is called diffusion, and if the molecule is uncharged, it is called non-ionic diffusion. In a population of drug molecules, the probability that during unit time any drug molecule will move across a boundary is directly proportional to the number of molecules crossing that boundary and therefore to the drug concentration.

Multiple Dose Administration: When a drug is given repeatedly at intervals shorter than those required to eliminate the drug of previously administered dose.

pH Partitioning Effect: This effect is of fundamental importance in gastro-intestinal absorption. The gastrointestinal tract is separated from the blood-stream by one layer of epithelial cells lining the lumen and by the walls of the blood capillaries at the base of the epithelial cells. The walls of the epithelial cells behave like lipid membranes, through which many drugs pass by a passive transport process. The rate of this process depends on the lipid solubility of the drug and especially on its oil/water partition coefficient.

Pharmacokinetics: The study of the changes in drug concentration of the drug product and changes of concentration of a drug and/or its metabolite(s) in the human or animal body following administration, or the changes of drug concentration in the different body fluids and tissues in the dynamic system of liberation, absorption, distribution, body storage, tissue binding metabolism, and excretion.

Potency: The potency of a drug is the reciprocal of dose. Potency generally has no other utility other than to provide a means of comparing the relative activities of drugs in a series.

Protein (or Tissue) Binding: The phenomenon which occurs when a drug combines with plasma protein (particularly albumin) or tissue protein to form a reversible complex. Protein binding is essentially non-specific and depends on the drug's affinity to the protein molecule, the number of protein binding sites, protein and drug concentration. Drugs can be displaced from protein binding by other compounds having higher affinity for the binding sites.

Receptor: A site in the biophase of the host being treated to which drug molecules can be bound. A receptor (substrate) is usually protein or proteinaceous material.

Renal Clearance: The hypothetical plasma volume in ml. (volume of distribution) of the parent drug which is cleared in one second by way of the kidney.

Selectivity: Despite the potential most drugs have for eliciting multiple effects, one effect is generally more readily elicitable than another. This differential responsiveness is usually considered to be a property of the drug, but it is also a property of the constitution and biodynamics of the recipient subject, such as the predilection of iodine for the thyroid.

Single Dose Administration: The next dose of the same drug is administered only after the drug of the previous dose is completely eliminated from the body. ·

Structural Nonspecific Drugs: Drug compounds whose pharmacological action is not directly dependent on chemical structure. They have no functional groups, are highly lipophilic, do not react easily, and act by physiochemical processes. Examples include ether, nitrous oxide, halothane, phenol, ethyl alcohol and acetone.

Structural Specific Drugs: Drug compounds whose pharmacological action results primarily from their chemical structure. They have functional groups, and combine to the three-dimensional structure of receptors in the biophase. Examples include antibiotics, sulfonamides, glycosides, anti-metabolites, anti-convulsants, among others.

Systemic Effect: The result obtained when the drug released from the drug product enters the blood and/or lymphatic systems and is distributed within the body or several organ systems, regardless of the site and route of administration.

Therapeutic Index: Used to designate a quantitative statement of the selectivity of a drug when a therapeutic and an untoward effect are being considered. If the untoward effect is designated as T and the therapeutic effect as E, the therapeutic index may be defined as TD_{50}/ED_{50} or a similar ratio at some other arbitrary levels of response.

Tolerance: A diminution in responsiveness as use of the drug continues. The consequence of tolerance is an increase in the dose requirement. It may be due to an increase in the rate of elimination of drug, to reflex or other compensatory homeostatic adjustments, to exhaustion of the effector system or depletion of mediators, to the development of immunity, or to other mechanisms. Tolerance may be gradual, requiring many doses and days to months to develop, or acute, requiring only the first or a few doses and only minutes to hours to develop. Acute tolerance is called tachyphylaxis.

Total Clearance: The clearance of the hypothetical plasma volume in milliliters (volume of distribution) of a drug per unit time due to excretion via kidney, liver, lung, and skin.

Tubular Reabsorption: The phenomenon that occurs when drugs filtered through the glomeruli are reabsorbed from the tubuli into systemic circulation.

Vehicle(s): Additive(s) which are necessary in formulating a dosage form from the drug. They are chemically inert and usually do not have any pharmacological effect in the dose used. Vehicle substances are used to produce, from a relatively small amount of drug, a dosage form of the desired strength, volume, form or consistency suitable for administration.

Volume of Distribution: A hypothetical volume of body fluid that would be required to dissolve the total amount of drug at the same concentration as that found in the blood.

TABLE 23. Mathematical Formulae and Concepts in Therapeutic Drug Monitoring

1.   HENDERSON-HASSELBALCH EQUATIONS - WEAK ACIDS
   (a)   Weak acid (HA) ionizes according to:
$$HA + H_2O = H_3O^+ + A^-$$
   (b)   The dissociation constant is given as:
$$K_a = \frac{[H_3O^+]\,[A^-]}{[HA]}$$
   K_a = Dissociation Constant
   A^- = Molar Concentration of the Acidic Anion
   H_3O^+ = Molar Concentration of the Hydronium Ion
   HA = Molar Concentration of the Undissociated Acid
   (c)   Henderson-Hasselbalch equation is calculated from
   (b) and becomes:
$$pH = \log \frac{[A^-]}{[HA]} + pK_a$$

2.   HENDERSON-HASSELBALCH EQUATIONS - WEAK BASES
   (a)   Weak base (BH$^+$) ionizes according to:
$$BH^+ + H_2O = H_3O^+ + B$$
   (b)   Henderson-Hasselbalch equation is calculated as
   in weak acid and becomes:
$$pH = \log \frac{[B]}{[BH^+]} + pK_a$$

3.   PERCENTAGE OF IONIZATION FOR WEAK ACID
$$\% \text{ Ionization (acid)} = \frac{100}{1 + \text{antilog} \;\;(pK_a\text{-}pH)}$$

   At 50% ionization, $pK_a = pH$

4.   PERCENTAGE OF IONIZATION FOR WEAK BASE
$$\% \text{ Ionization (base)} = \frac{100}{1 + \text{antilog} \;\;(pH\text{-}pK_a)}$$

5.   RITSCHEL'S THEORETICAL EQUILIBRIUM RATIOS
   (a)   Weak Acids:
$$R_a = \frac{1 + \text{antilog} \,(pH_x\text{-}pK_a)}{1 + \text{antilog} \,(pH_p\text{-}pK_a)}$$

   (b)   Weak bases:
$$R_b = \frac{1 + \text{antilog} \,(pK_a\text{-}pH_x)}{1 + \text{antilog} \,(pK_a\text{-}pH_p)}$$

R_a = Concentration Ratio between any compartment and plasma for weak acids

R_b = Concentration Ratio between any compartment and plasma for weak bases

Cx = Concentration in the extra vascular compartment (milk, cerebrospinal fluid, sweat, rectal fluid, stomach fluid, intestinal fluid)

Cp = Concentration in plasma

pH_x = pH of Extravascular Compartment

pH_p = pH of plasma (7.4)

6. CALCULATION OF PROTEIN BINDING
   (a) Reversible process as follows:

   $$(D) + (P) \underset{K_d}{\overset{K_a}{\rightleftarrows}} (D\text{-}P)$$

   (D) = Concentration of Free Drug (moles/liter)

   (P) = Concentration of Free Protein (moles/liter)

   (D-P) = Drug-protein Complex Concentration

   K_a = Association Constant

   K_d = Dissociation Constant = $1/K_a$

   (b) Association Constant is expressed as follows:

   $$K_a = \frac{(D\text{-}P)}{(D)\,(P)}$$

   (c) Quantity of binding (r) is defined as moles of drug bound divided by total moles of protein present:

   $$r = \frac{[D\text{-}P]}{[D\text{-}P] + [P]}$$

   (d) Quantity of total binding ($r$total) for more than one binding site:

   $$r\text{total} = \frac{N\,K_a(D)}{1 + K_a(D)}$$

   N = number of binding sites

7. GLOMERULAR FILTRATION OF DRUGS (For drugs not bound to plasma proteins)

   t = Time   F = Cp · GFR (mg/min)

   F = Amount of drug filtered through a glomeruli (mg/min)

   Cp = Drug Concentration in plasma (mg/ml)

   GFR = Glomerular Filtration Rate = renal clearance (ml/min)

8. AMOUNT OF DRUG FILTERED THROUGH GLOMERULI

$$F = [(1-p) \cdot Cp] \cdot Cl_{creat} \text{ (mg/min)}$$

F = Amount of drug filtered through glomeruli (mg/min)

Cp = Concentration of drug in plasma (mg/ml)

p = Fraction of drug bound to protein

Cl_{creat} = Creatinine Clearance (ml/min)

9. RENAL CLEARANCE (NO PROTEIN BINDING)

Volume of blood that is cleared of the drug during one minute by way of the kidneys is described as follows:

$$Cl_{ren} = \frac{(Cu)\,(V)}{Cp} \text{ (ml/min)}$$

Cl_{ren} = Renal Clearance

Cu = Concentration of drug in urine (mg/ml)

V = Volume of urine excreted (ml/min)

Cp = Concentration of drug in plasma (mg/ml),
     at midpoint of urine collection,

10. CREATININE CLEARANCE

Determined by collecting urine for exactly 24 hours and
taking blood sample at midpoint, and calculated is as follows:

$$Cl_{creat} = \frac{Cu \cdot V \cdot 100}{Cp \cdot 1440} \text{ (ml/min)}$$

Cl_{creat} = Observed Creatinine Clearance (ml/min)

Cu = Creatinine Concentration in urine (mg/ml)

V = Volume of urine excreted in 24 hours (ml)

Cp = Creatinine Concentration in serum (mg/100 ml),
     at midpoint in urine collection

11. RENAL CLEARANCE (PROTEIN BINDING OF DRUG)

$$Cl_{ren.\,corr.} = \frac{Cu \cdot V}{(1-p) \cdot Cp}$$

$Cl_{ren.\,corr.}$ = Corrected Renal Clearance (ml/min)

p = Fraction of drugs bound to protein

Cu = Concentration of drug urine (mg/ml)

V = Volume of urine excreted (ml/min)

Cp = Concentration of drug in plasma (mg/ml), at
     midpoint of urine collection

12. AMOUNT OF DRUG EXCRETED

$$E = Cu \cdot V \text{ (mg/min)}$$

E = Amount of drug excreted via kidney (mg/ml)

Cu = Concentration of drug in urine (mg/ml)

V = Volume of urine excreted (ml/min)

13. AMOUNT DRUG REABSORBED

The amount of drug filtered through the glomerulus but
reabsorbed from the tubuli into the bloodstream is calculated as follows:

RA = Filtered drug - Excreted drug

$RA = (Cl_{creat} \ [(1-p)Cp] - (CuV) \ (mg/min)$

RA = Amount of Drug Reabsorbed (mg/min)

14. EXCRETION RATIO

The excretion ratio (E-R) considers the extent of protein binding of a particular drug.
It is the fraction of free drug removed by glomerular filtration during circulation through the kidneys :

$$E\text{-}R = \frac{Cl_{ren \, corr}}{Cl_{creat}}$$

15. TOTAL CLEARANCE

The total clearance characterizes the clearing of 2
given drugs' hypothetical plasma volume, including all
pathways of excretion and metabolism.

For the open one compartment model the total clearance is determined:

$$Cl_{tot} = \frac{k_e \cdot V_d}{60} \ (ml/min)$$

Cl_{tot} = Total Clearance (ml/min)
k_e = Overall Elimination Rate Constant (hr^{-1})
V_d = Volume of Distribution (ml)

For the open two compartment model:

$$Cl_{tot} = \frac{k_r \cdot V_c}{60} \ (ml/min)$$

k_r = Elemination rate constant (hr^{-1})
V_c = Volume of central compartment (ml)

16. EXTRARENAL CLEARANCE

The extrarenal clearance is calculated as such:

$$Cl_{extraren} = Cl_{tot} - Cl_{ren \, corr} \ (ml/min)$$

Since the excretion of a drug into the extravascular compartments (cerebro - spinal fluid, sweat,
stomach fluids, intestinal fluids) and bile are not increased in the renal clearance, but elevated in the
total clearance determinations, the extrarenal clearance may give a positive indication of the degree of
metabolism or biliary excretion of a given drug compound, providing other factors such as lung and
salivarily clearance contributes little to the extrarenal clearance.

17.   INULIN CLEARANCE

The use of the polysaccharide, inulin, for measuring glomeruler filtration rate (GFR) is usually not regarded as a routine clinical test. Since inulin is not normally present in the plasma, it must be introduced at a proper concentration to allow its clearance by the kidney to be measured. This is normally done by giving a sufficient quantity as a priming dose by intravenous interjection to produce a constant plasma level and then maintain this level throughout the test period by a slow infusion of a solution. After the priming dose of inulin and satisfactory plasma levels have been reached, after about one-half hour the bladder is emptied and subsequently urine is collected in three accurately timed specimens of about 20 minutes each. Blood specimens are withdrawn at the beginning and at the end of the urine collection period. Simultaneously measurement of the plasma inulin and the quantity of urine excreted at a given time then supplies the data necessary to calculate the clearance as follows:

$$Inulin_{Cl}= \frac{(Inulin_u)\ (V)}{Inulin_B}$$

$Inulin_C$ = Clearance of Inulin (ml/min)
$Inulin_u$ = Urinary Inulin (mg/100 ml)
$Inulin_B$ = Blood Inulin (mg/100 ml)
V = Volume of Urine (ml/min)

18.   FICK'S LAW OF DIFFUSION OF DRUG THROUGH MEMBRANES

$$\frac{dQ}{dt}= \frac{DA\ (C_1-C_2)}{x}$$

Q = The net quantity of drug transferred across membrane

C_1 = The concentration on one side of membrane
C_2 = The concentration on the reverse side of membrane

x = Thickness of one membrane
A = Area
D = Diffusion Coefficient, related to permeability

It is normally customary to combine the membrane factors into a single constant, called a Permeability Constant or Coefficient, P, so that $P = D/x(A)$. The Rate of Net Transport (diffusion) across one membrane then becomes:

$$\frac{dQ}{dt} =P(C_1-C_2)$$

Equilibrium is defined as that state in which $C_1 = C_2$

19. NERNST EQUATION

At electrochemical equilibrium at body temperature (37°C),
ionized drug molecules will be distributed according to the following equation:

$$\pm \log \frac{C_o}{C_i} = \frac{ZE}{61}$$

C_o = Molar extracellular concentration
C_i = Molar intracellular concentration
Z = Number of Charols per molecule
E = Membrane potential, millivolts
Log C_o/C_i is positive when the molecule is negatively charged and negative when the molecule is
positively charged.

20. VOLUME OF DISTRIBUTION

$$V_d = \frac{Q}{C_p}$$

V_d = Volume of distribution (liters)
Q = Quantity of drug (milligrams)
C_p = Concentration of drug in the plasma in milligrams

21. STOMACH EMPTYING RATE

Transit time in the stomach may have a very important
effect on drug absorption; it varies with individuals
and with the amount and osmotic pressure of stomach
contents and may provide useful data
in overdose cases as to the amount of drug
and time injected. In general, it appears to
follow a pseudo first-order process, in
accordance with the equation:

$$\frac{W_t}{W_o} = e^{-kt}$$

W_0 = Initial weight of stomach contents
W_t = Weight of Stomach Contents at time (t)
k = Emptying rate constant

TABLE 24. Relative Human Tissue pH Values

Tissue/Location	Range pH Values
Bile	5.6-8.0
Bile, in liver	7.5-7.8
Bile, in Gall Bladder	6.6-6.7
Blood, arterial	7.35-7.45
Blood, venous	7.32-7.42
Cerebrospinal fluid	7.32-7.37
Gastric fluid	Men: 1.85-1.93
	Women:2.48-2.63
	Children: 0.8-7.8
Milk	6.6-7.0
Pancreatic fluid	7.5-8.8
Saliva, adults	5.8-7.1
Saliva, children	6.4-8.2
Sweat	4.0-6.8
Urine, adults	4.8-7.5
Urine, children	5.1-7.2
Feces, adults	5.9-8.5
Feces, children	4.6-5.2
Stomach	1.0-3.5
Duodenum	6.5-7.6
Jejunum	6.3-7.3
Ileum	7.4-7.6
Colon	7.9-8.0
Rectum	7.7-7.9
Plasma	7.40-7.45

TABLE 25. Volume and Composition of Human Blood Plasma and Other Physiological Fluids

Fluid	Average Volume (ml/24 hours)	Electrolyte Concentrations (mEq/liter)			
		Na^+	k^+	Cl^-	HCO_3^-
Blood Plasma	-	135-145	3.8-5.2	98-108	25-29
Gastric Juice	2500	31-90	4.0-12	50-130	0
Bile	700-1000	134-156	4.0-6.5	83-110	38
Pancreatic Fluid	>1000	113-153	2.6-7.4	53-97	110
Feces	100	<10	<10	<15	<15
Sweat	500-4000	30-70	0-5	30-70	0

TABLE 26. Age Versus Renal Clearance (Cl$_{ren}$)

Age Group	Cl$_{ren}$ (ml/min/1.73m^2)
1-10 Days	15-45
1 Month	30-60
6 Months	50-100
1 Year	80-120
1-70 Years	80-140
70-80 Years	70-110
80-90 Years	45-85

TABLE 27. Excretion Patterns of Various Drug Substances

Pathway of Excretion	Mechanism	Drug Examples
Urine	Glomerular filtration, active tubular secretion	Most drugs in free (nonprotein bound) form: Salicylic acid, PAH, N'-methylnicotinamide, PAB, penicillin, acetylsulfonamides, organic mercuric diuretics, chlorothiazide
Bile	Active transport, passive diffusion, pinocytosis	Quarternary ammonium compounds, strychnine, quinine, digitoxin, penicillin, streptomycin, tetracyclines
Intestines	Passive diffusion and biliary secretion	Ionized organic acids
Saliva	Passive diffusion and active transport	Penicillin, tetracyclines, thiamine, desoxycholate, ethanol, ether
Lung	Passive diffusion	Camphor, ammonium chloride, iodides, sodium bicarbonate
Sweat	Passive diffusion	Weak organic acids and bases, thiamine
Milk	Passive diffusion and active transport	Primarily weak organic bases, less weak acids, anesthetics, anti-coagulants, erythromycin and other anti-biotics

TABLE 28. Drugs Excreted into urine by Renal Absorption

Increased Rate of Excretion in Acidic Urine	Increased Rate of Excretion in Alkaline Urine
Amphetamine	Acetazolamide
Chloroquine	Amino acids
Codeine	Barbiturates
Imipramine	Nalidixic acid
Mecamylamine	Phenylbutazone
Meperidine	Probenecid
Morphine	Salicylic acid
Nicotine	Sulfonamides
Procaine	
Quinidine	
Quinine	

Table 29. Drugs Altering Urinary pH

Acidosis	Alkalosis
Acetazolamide	Antacids
Ammonium Chloride	Calcium Carbonate
Ascorbic acid	Diuretics, Mercurial
Aspirin	Diuretics, Thiazides
Dimercaprol	Sodium Bicarbonate
Phenformin HCl	Sodium Glutamate
Salicylates	

Table 30. Drugs Secreted by Active Transport into the Tubuli

Acids	Bases
Amino acids	Dihydromorphine
p-Aminohippuric acid	Choline
Acetazolamide	Dopamine
Furosemide	Histamine
Indomethacin	N'-Methylnicotinamide
Penicillins	Neostigmine
Phenol Red	Quinine
Phenylbutazone	Tetraethylammonium
Salicylates	
Thiazides	

Table 31. Rates of Entry and Degrees of Ionization of Selected Drugs in CSF at ph7.4

Drug	% Binding to PlasmaProtein	pKa[1]	% Unionized at pH 7.4	Permeability Constant (Pmin $^{-1}$) ±S.E.
	Drugs Mainly Ionized at pH 7.4			
5-Sulfosalicylic acid	22	(strong)	0	<0.0001
N[1]-Methylnicotinamide	<10	(strong)	0	0.0005±0.00006
5-Nitrosalicyclic acid	42	2.3	0.001	0.001±0.0001
Salicyclic Acid	40	3.0	0.004	0.006±0.0004
Quinine	76	8.4	9.09	0.078±0.0061
	Drugs Mainly Unionized at pH 7.4			
Barbital	<2	7.5	55.7	0.026±0.0022
Thiopental	75	7.6	61.3	0.50±0.051
Pentobarbital	40	8.1	83.4	0.17±0.014
Aminopyrine	20	5.0	99.6	0.25±0.020
Aniline	15	4.6	99.8	0.40±0.042
Sulfaguanidine	6	>10.0	>99.8	0.003±0.0002
Antipyrine	8	1.4	>99.8	0.12±0.013

[1]Dissociation constant (pKa) of both acids and bases expressed as negative log of the acidic dissociation constant.

TABLE 32. Drug Type and Sequence of Metabolic Transformations

Drug Chemical Class/ Functional Group	Type and Sequence of Metabolic Transformation
Aromatic rings	Hydroxylation
Aliphatic Hydroxyl group	Chain oxidation, glucuronic acid or sulfate conjugation
Aromatic Hydroxyl group	Ring hydroxylation, glucuronic acid or sulfate conjugation, or methylation
Aliphatic Carboxyl group	Glucuronic acid or amino acid conjugation
Aromatic Carboxyl group	Ring hydroxylation, amino acid or glucuronic conjugation
Aliphatic primary amines	Deamination, methylation
Aromatic primary amines	Ring hydroxylation, acetylation, or glucuronic acid conjugation, or methylation and sulfate conjugation
Secondary and tertiary amines	Dealkylation, methylation
Sulhydryl group	Glucuronic acid conjugation, methylation or oxidation

TABLE 33. Dissociation Constants of Selected Weak Acids (pKa)

Acid	pKa	Acid	pKa
Acetic	4.76	Phosphoric	K_1 2.12
Acetylsalicylic	3.49		K_2 7.21
Barbituric	7.97		K_3 12.32
Benzoic	4.20	Phthalic	K_1 2.90
Boric	9.24		K_2 5.51
Carbonic	K_1 6.37	Picric	0.38
	K_2 10.33	Propionic	4.87
Citric	K_1 3.08	Saccharin	1.60
	K_2 4.74		
	K_3 5.40	Salicylic	2.97
Fumaric	K_1 3.03	Secobarbital	7.90
	K_2 4.38	Succinic	K_1 4.19
Hypochlorous	7.43		K_2 5.63
Lactic	3.86	Sulphuric	K_1 -
Mandelic	3.37		K_2 1.92
Nitrous	3.35	Tartaric	K_1 3.02
Oxalic	K_1 1.26		K_2 4.36
	K_2 4.28	Thiopental	7.60
Phenobarbital	7.41	Trichloroacetic	0.89
Phenylbutazone	4.38	Valeric	4.81
Phenol	10.00	Valproic	4.58

TABLE 34. Dissociation Constants of Selected Weak Bases (pKb)

Base	pKb	Base	pKb
Acetanilid	13.68	Pilocarpine	K_1 7.2
Ammonium Hydroxide	4.74		K_2 12.7
Atropine	4.35	Piperazine	K_1 4.19
Benzocaine	11.22		K_2 8.43
Caffeine	13.39	Procaine	5.15
Calcium Hydroxide	K_1 -	Pyridine	8.85
	K_2 1.40		
Chlordiazepoxide	9.24	Quinidine	K_1 5.43
Cocaine	5.59		K_2 10.00
Codeine	6.05	Quinine	K_1 5.96
Diazepam	10.59		K_2 9.87
Ephedrine	4.64	Reserpine	7.4
Ethylenediamine	4.07	Strychnine	K_1 6.0
Morphine	6.13		K_2 11.7
Noscapine	7.82	Theobromine	13.32
Papaverine	8.10	Theophylline	13.34
Physostigmine	K_1 6.12	Urea	13.82
	K_2 12.24		

TABLE 35. Psychotropic Drug Classification

DRUG GROUPS	SYNONYMS	WORKING DEFINITION	SUB-GROUPS	EXAMPLES
NEUROLEPTICS:	Major Tranquilizers Neuroplegics Psychoplegics Psycholeptics Antipsychotics	Non-hypnotic drugs with antipsychotic effects	Phenothiazine Derivatives .... Benzoquinolizine Derivatives .... Thioxanthene Derivatives .... Butyrophenone Derivatives .... Rauwolfia Alkaloids .... Other:	Chlorpromazine Thioridazine Fluphenazine Tetrabenazine Chlorprothixene Haloperidol Reserpine
			Benzodiazepines Derivatives .... Glycol Derivatives	Chlordiazepoxide Oxazepam Meprobamate Phenaglycodol
ANXIOLYTICS:	Antianxiety Drugs Minor Tranquilizers Sedatives	Non-hypnotic drugs with antianxiety effects but without antipsychotic effects	Carbinols .... Diphenylmethane Derivatives .... Barbiturates .... MAO-Inhibitors	Phenprobamate Methaqualone Hydroxine Phenobarbital Amobarbital Isocarboxazid Nialamide Phenelzine
ANTI-DEPRESSANTS:	Thymoleptics Thymoanaleptics Psychoanaleptics Psychic Energizers	Drugs which elevate mood and relieve depression	Tricyclics .... Phenylethylamine Derivatives	Tranylcypromine Imipramine Desipramine Amitriptyline Protriptyline Amphetamine Methamphetamine

TABLE 35. (Cont.)

Category	Subtypes	Description	Subgroups / Examples
STIMULANTS:	Psychoanaleptics Psychotonics Analeptics Psychomotor Stimulants	Drugs which accelerate psychomotor function and activity and improve performance under conditions of fatigue	Other: .... Phenmetrazine Methylphenidate Pipradol
PSYCHO-TOMIMETICS:	Psycholytics Psychodysleptics Hallucinogenics Psychedelics Eidetics	Drugs producing alteration in consciousness, characterized by perceptual and emotional changes without disorientation	Phenylethylamine Derivatives .... Mescaline Indole-alkaloids .... LSD Psilocybin Tryptamine Derivatives Piperidine Derivatives .... Ditran Phencyclidine
HYPNOTICS:	Soporifics Somnifacients	Psycholeptics with sleep-inducing and sleep-sustaining effects	Barbiturates .... Secobarbital Pentobarbital Non-Barbiturates .... Glutethimide Other: Ethinamate

[1]Reproduced with permission of Dr. Alice Leeds, from Psychopermacology Bulletin, 14(3):2, 1978

Table 36. Effects of Drugs on Activity of Liver Microsomal Enzymes

Type of Drug	Stimulate Activity	No Effect	Depress Activity
Anesthetics	Ether, Chloroform, Nitrous oxide	Divinyl ether, Halothane	Ether
Hypnotics and sedatives	Barbiturates, Glutethimide, Urethane, Chlorobutanol, Methyprylone	Ethinamate, Thaliodomide, Paraldehyde	Ethanol, Chloral-hydrate, Chloralose
Tranquilizers	Phenaglycodol, Meprobamate, Chlorpromazine, Triflupro-mazine	Promazine, Chlordiazepoxide	Meprobamate
Anticonvulsants	Primidone, Phenytoin, Paramethadione	Trimethadione	Phenytoin
Muscle relaxants	Carisoprodol, Mephenesin	Zoxazolamine	
Analeptics and psycho-motor stimulants	Bemigride, Imipramine, Iproniazid	Amphetamine	Pheniprazine, Iproniazid
Analgesics	Phenylbutazone, Amino-pyrine, Meperidine		Morphine (and congeners)
Antihistamines	Diphenhydramine, Chlor-cyclizine		
Sulphonamides and Antibiotics	Tolbutamide	Sulphanilamide	Chloramphenicol
Steroids	Androgens, Adrenocorti-coids		Estrogens, Progesterone
Polycyclic hydrocarbons	3,4-Benzpyrene, 3-Methyl-cholanthrene, 1,2:5,6-Dibenzanthracene		
Insecticides	Chlorinated hydrocarbons (DDT, dieldron, aldrin)	Pyrethrum, Piperonyl butoxide	

TABLE 37. Urinary Excretion of Drugs

Drug	Percentage of Dose
Sulfonamides	90-100
Penicillin	60-90
Salicylate	70-90
p-Aminosalicylic acid	65-90
Morphine	85-95
Streptomycin	75
Tetracycline	50-60
Heparin	20-50
Phenobarbital	15-25
Atropine	13
Ethanol	Less than 5
Procaine	0

[1]Reproduced from Clin. Pharmacokinetics *1*:351-72, 1976, with permission of Dr. M. Kristensen and Publisher ADIS Press, Australia.

Table 38. Normal Renal Functions in Man

Cardiac output at rest	5,600 ml/min
Renal blood flow (1/4 of cardiac output	1,400 ml/min
Renal plasma flow (hematocrit-50 percent)	700 ml/min
Glomerular filtration rate (1/5 renal plasma flow)	140 ml/min or 17) liters per day
Urinary output	1-1.5 ml/min or 1.5-2 liters per day
Tubular absorption of filtered fluid	99.9 percent
Na^+ in plasma	145 mEq/liter
Total Na^+ filtered in glomeruli	26 Eq/day or 1,500 g/day NaCl
Total Na^+ excreted in urine	10 g/day NaCl
Na^+ reabsorbed	99 percent

Table 39. Biliary Excretion of Various Drugs

Drugs	Species	Percent of Administered Dose Excreted in Bile			Time in Hrs.
		Free form	Metabol. Form	Total	
Organic acids:					
Sulfobromophthalein	Man	13	48	61	2
Iopanoic acid	Cat	---	75	75	18
Acetyliopanoic acid		---	---	30	18
Sulfadimethoxine	Rat	---	11	11	24
Penicillin-G	Dog	---	---	9	24
Methicillin		---	---	22	24
Chlorothiazide		---	---	41	4
Hydrochlorothiazide		---	---	4	1
p-aminobenzoic acid	Rat	---	---	3	24
o-aminobenzoic acid		---	---	5	24
Salicyclic acid		---	2	2	24
Organic bases:					
Morphine	Dog	0.2	39.8	40	12
	Monkey	0.1	11.9	12	4
Methadone	Rat	1.5	7.5	9	24
Epinephrine		---	10	10	7
Isoproterenol		---	38	38	8
Atropine		---	50	50	4
Steroids and hormones:					
Estradiol	Man	---	50	50	48
Progesterone		---	36	36	
Testosterone		---	13	13	1
Corticosterone		---	25	25	
Cortisone		---	3	3	
Thyroxine		---	---	10	95
Others:					
Digitoxin	Dog	3	36	39	8
Digoxin		1	14	15	108
Glutethimide	Rat	3	57	60	15
Amitriptyline		---	50	50	6
Coumarin		---	50	50	24

TABLE 40. Variation Between Plasma Levels of Phenytoin and Phenobarbital as an Index of Compliance

Drug	Variation (%)	Frequency (%)			
		Sample No. 2 vs. 1	Sample No. 3 vs. 2	Sample No. 4 vs. 3	
Phenytoin	10	29 (8/28)	0 (0/19)	8 (1/12)	
	10-20	11 (3/28)	16 (3/19)	17 (2/12)	
	20	61 (17/28)	84 (16/19)	74 (9/12)	
	Mean variation ± S.E.	45.3 ± 8.7%	209 ± 25%	197 ± 22%	
	Median variation	24.7%	57.0%	42.0%	
Phenobarbital	10	13 (3/24)	25 (3/12)	0 (0/12)	
	10-20	17 (4/24)	33 (4/12)	17 (2/12)	
	20	71 (17/24)	42 (5/12)	83 (10/12)	
	Mean variation ± S.E.	18.3 ± 3.8%	59.1 ± 8.6%	67.5 ± 8.8%	
	Median variation	28.3%	17.4%	94.7%	

Patients included are those from whom no change in anticonvulsant dose was made during the period of observation. Number of patients receiving the drug (denominator) and showing a given percent variation (numerator) is shown in parenthesis.

Variation is calculated as $\dfrac{a - b}{a}$ (100) = % Variation. Frequency (%) represents the percent of patients for a given variation.

- From Wilson, J.T. and Wilkinson, G.R. Delivery of Anticonvulsant Drug Therapy in Epileptic Patients Assessed by Plasma Level Analyses. Neurology (Minneapolis) 24:614-623, 1974.

TABLE 41. Pharmacokinetic Data on Selected Therapeutically Monitored Drugs

Drug	Biological Half-Life (t½), hrs.	Drug Excreted Unchanged in Urine, %	Protein Binding, %	pKa
Acetaminophen	1-4	1-4	20-50	9.5
Amikacin	2-3	94	0	
Amobarbital	13-45	< 1.0	34	7.94
Amphetamine	7-140 (urine pH > 6.6)	67.0-73.0	-	
	18-34.0 (urine pH < 6.6)	17.0-43.0	-	
Amitriptyline	15-25	1-2	80-95	
Aprobarbital	0.5-1.5 days	13.7	50-75	
Barbital	2.4-3.3 days	80.0-90.0	-	7.91
Carbamazepine	10-28	< 10.0	60-73	
Carbamazepine-10,11-epoxide	5-16	1-3	-	
Chlordiazepoxide	5-20	< 5.0	80-90	
Chlorpromazine	16-30	< 1.0	95-98	
Clonazepam	13-46		40-70	10.5
Desipramine	12-24	5-15	90	---
Diazepam	20-40	< 1.0	96	3.4
Desmethyldiazepam	60-95	10	---	---
Digitoxin	5-8 days	< 1.0	97	---
Digoxin	0.7-2.0 days	60-90	23	---
Dimethadione	240		0	
Disopyramide	4-10	45-72		50
Doxepin	> 12		80-90	
Ethosuximide	60	19	0	9.3
Ethotoin	15-25	---	---	---
Flurazepam	24-48			---
N-Desalkyl-flurazepam	> 24			---
Gentamicin	2-4	50-90	10	---
Glutethimide	5-22	up to 5.0	50	
Haloperidol	13-36	< 10	> 70	---
Imipramine	8-16	< 10	90-98	---
Indomethacin	2-8	10-20	90	4.5
Isoniazid	1.0-2.0, rapid acetylator	37	15-35	10.77
	3.0-3.8, slow acetylator	66	---	---
Lidocaine	1-2	2-10	66	7.86
Monoethylglycine-xylidide	2.4	60-75	60	
Lithium	10-24	89-98	0	6.8
Meperidine	1.5-4.0	< 5.0	40	---
Mephenytoin	Not established	---	20-50	---
Mephobarbital	1-3	< 1.0	40-60	7.8
Methadone	15-30	16-30	87	8.62
Methotrexate	1-1.5 Triphasic: 0.8, 3.5, 28	50-100 (dose dependent)	50-70	4.3, 5.5
Methsuximide	1.2-1.6	---	0	---
Normethsuximide	28-36	---	0	---
Nortriptyline	18-93	0.5-4.0	92-96	
Paramethadione	24-72	< 1.0	0	---
5-ethyl-5-methyl-2, 4-oxazolidine-dione	150-300	30-80	0	---
Pentobarbital	40-50	0	35-70	8.1
Phenobarbital	50-120	13-35	45-50	7.41

TABLE 41. (cont.)

Drug	Biological Half-Life (t$_{1/2}$), hrs.	Drug Excreted Unchanged in Urine, %	Protein Binding, %	pKa
Phensuximide	6-8.5	---	0	---
Phenytoin	18-22	< 1.0	88	8.3
Primidone	6-8	20-40	0-30	> 13
Phenylethyl-malonamide	24-48	10-30	---	---
Procainamide	2.0-4.0	40-55	15	9.2
N-acetyl-procainamide	3.0-6.0	30-40	---	---
Propranolol	3.0-6.0	0	93	9.45
4-hydroxy-propranolol	4.0-8.0	15-60	---	---
Quinidine Gluconate	3.0-16.0	0	---	5.4
Quinidine Sulfate	7.2	15	82	8.8
Salicylic acid	0.5-30 (dose dependent)	5-40 (dose dependent)	50-90	2.97
Sulfadiazine	10-20	50-70	45	6.4
Sulfadimethoxine	60-70	58	99	6.1
Sulfamethazine	7.0	10-30	80	7.4
Sulfamethoxazole	8-14	30	68	6.0
Sulfisoxazole	6.0	53	86	4.9
Theophylline	3-8	10	60	8.6
Tobramycin	3-5	95	10	---
Tolbutamide	3.5-8.0	10-25	50-80	---
Trimethadione	16-20	2-4	0	---
Valproic acid	7-15	< 7.0	90-100	4.95
Warfarin	29-70	< 1.0	97-100	5.05

Newton, D.W. and Kluza, R.B. pKa values of Medicinal Compounds in Pharmacy Practice. *Drg Int. and Clin Pharm.* 12:Sept. 1978.

TABLE 42. Correlation Between Type of Epilepsy, Drugs Likely to be Effective, and Therapeutic Ranges

Type of Epilepsy	Drug Likely to be Effective	Therapeutic Range in Serum, mg/liter
Absences (petit mal)	Ethosuximide	40-100
	Methsuximide	10-40 (as Normethsuximide)
	Trimethadione	200-800 (as Dimethadione)
Myoclonic seizures	Valproic acid	60-130
	Diazepam	0.05-0.20
	Clonazepam	5-70 ng/ml
Convulsive seizures	Phenobarbital	15-40
	Mephobarbital	5-15
	Primidone	5-12
	Carbamazepine	8-12
	Phenytoin	10-20

(Generalized encompasses Absences, Myoclonic seizures, and Convulsive seizures; Partial connects to Convulsive seizures.)

Adapted from Eadie (1976) with permission from Dr. M.J. Eadie and The ADIS Press.

REFERENCES

1. **AACC, Theraputic Drug Monitoring Continuing Education and Quality Control Program.** Year 1 testing program. American Association for Clinical Chemistry, Washington, D.C. 1980

2. **Abramson EA, Arky RA.** Role of beta-adrenergic receptors in counterregulation to insulin-induced hypoglycemia. Diabetes 1968; 17:141

3. **Acocella G,** et al. Kinetics of rifampicin and isoniazid administered alone and in combination to normal subjects and patients with liver disease. Gut 1972; 13:47-53

4. **Adamson RH.** Metabolism of anticancer agents in man. Ann NY Acad Sci 1971; 179:432-41

5. **Aderhold RM, Muniz CE.** Acute psychosis with amitriptyline and furazolidone (Letter). JAMA 1970; 213:2080

6. **Albert KS,** et al. Pharmacokinetics of orally administered acetaminophen in man. J Pharmacokin Biopharm 1974a; 2:381-93

7. **Albert KS,** et al. Bioavailability studies of acetaminophen and nitrofurantoin. J Clin Pharmacol 1974b; 14:264-70

8. **Alexanderson B.** Pharmacokinetics of desmethylimipramine and nortriptyline in man after single and multiple oral doses - A cross-over study. Eur J Clin Pharmacol 1972; 5:1-10

9. **Alexanderson B, Evans DAP, Sjoquist F.** Steady state plasma levels of nortriptyline therapy. British Med Journal 1971; 4:764-8

10. **Alvan G, Orme M.** Pharmicokinetics of indomethacin. Clin Pharmacol Ther 1975; 18:364-72

11. **Ambre JJ, Fischer LJ.** Identification and activity of the hydroxy metabolite that accumulates in the plasma of humans intoxicated with glutethimide. Drug Metab Digestion 1974; 2:151-8

12. **Amdisen A, Sjogren J.** Lithium absorption from sustained-release tablets (Duretter). Acta Pharmacol Suecica 1968; 5:465-72

13. **American Association for Clinical Chemistry.** "Therapuetic Drug Monitoring" - Continuing Education and Quality Control Year 1 - Testing Program, Washington, D.C. 1980

14. **American Hospital Formulary Service.** Imipramine 28: 16.04 (June) 1962. American Society of Hospital Pharmacies, Washington, D.C.

15. **American Hospital Formulary Service.** Sulfonamides 8:24 (Nov.) 1969. American Society of Hospital Pharmacists, Washington, D.C.

16. **AMA Drug Evaluations, ed.** AMA/DE-3 Chicago: American Medical Association. 1977

17. **Anggard E,** et al. Pharmacokinetic and clinical studies on amphetamine dependent subjects. Eur J Clin Pharmacol 1970; 3:3-11

18. **Anggard E,** et al. Amphetamine metabolism in amphetamine psychosis. Clin Pharmacol Ther 1973; 14: 870-80

19. **Annotations.** Propranolol. Lancet 1967; 1:939

20. **Anon.** Council on Drugs—Evaluation of a new antituberculous agent, Rifampin (Rifadin, Rimactane). JAMA 1972; 220:414

21. **Anon.** Drug interactions that can affect your patients. Patient Care (Nov.) 1967; 1:32

22. **Anon.** FDA approves lithium for manic depression. (Medical News) JAMA 1970; 212:558

23. **Anon.**Heavy drinking accelerates drugs' breakdown in the liver. (Medical News) JAMA 1968; 206:1709

24. **Anon.** New Drugs. 3rd ed. Chicago, IL: Council on Drugs of the American Medical Association. 1967. pp. 427-39

25. **Anon.** Methylphenidate (Ritalin). The Medical Letter 1969; 11:47

26. **Anon.** Stimulant augments antidepressant. (Medical News) JAMA 1969; 208:1616

27. **Antlitz AM, Awalt LF.** A double blind study of acetaminophen used in conjunction with oral anticoagulant therapy. Curr Ther Res 1969; 11: 360

28. **Antlitz AM** et al. Effect of butabarbital on orally administered anticoagulants. Curr Ther Res 1968; 10:70

29. **Antlitz AM,** et al. Potentiation of oral anticoagulant therapy by acetaminophen. Curr Ther Res 1968; 10:501

30. **Anton AH.** The effect of disease, drugs, and dilution on the binding of sulfonamides in human plasma. Clin Pharmacol Ther 1968; 9:561

31. **Anton AH, Solomen HM.** eds. Drug-Protein Binding. Ann NY Acad Sci 1973; 226

32. **Arena J.** Poisoning-Toxicology, Symptoms, Treatments. 3rd ed. Springfield IL: Charles C. Thomas. 1974

33. **Ariens AJ, Simonis AM, Van Rossum JM.** The Relation Between Stimulus and Effect. Mol Pharmacol 1964; 1:394

34. **Arnold K, Gerber N.** The rate of decline of diphenylhydantoin in human plasma. Clin Pharmacol Ther 1970; 11:121-34

35. **Asberg M,** et al. Relationship between plasma level and therapeutic effect on nortriptyline. Br Med J 1971; 3:331-4

36. **Atkinson AJ, Strong JM.** Effect of active drug metabolites on plasma-level response correlations. J Pharmacol Biopharmaceut 1977; 5:95

37. **Azarnoff DL, Hurwitz A.** Drug interactions. Pharmacol Physicians (Feb.) 1970; 4:1

38. **Baker L,** et al. Beta adrenergic blockage and juvenile diabetes: Acute studies and long-term therapeutic trial. J Pediat 1969; 75:19

39. **Balows A, Barker A.** A comparison of multitipped and conventional disc techniques for determining in vitro antibiotic sensitivity. Antibiotics Chemo. 1955; 5 (10): 551-4

40. **Barb RR, Wilbur RS.** Aspirin and gastrointestinal bleeding. An opinion. Calif Med 1969; 110:440

41. **Barr WH,** et al. Decrease of tetracycline absorption in man by sodium bicarbonate. Paper presented at the American Pharmaceutical Assoc. Annual Meeting, April 16, 1970

42. **Barrow MV,** et al. Salicylate hypoprothrombinemia in rheumatoid arthritis with liver disease. Arch Int Med 1967; 120:620

43. **Barry AL, Garcia F, Thrupp LD.** An improved method for testing the antibiotic susceptibility of rapidly growing pathogens. Am J Clin Pathol 1970; 53:149-58

44. **Baselt RC, Casarett LJ.** Urinary excretion of methadone in man. Clin Pharmacol Ther 1972; 13:64-70

45. **Bauer AW, Kirby WMM, Sherris JC, Turck M.** Antibiotic susceptibility testing by a standardized single disk method. Am J Clin Pathol 1966; 45:493-6

46. **Baylis EM,** et al. Influence of folic acid on blood-phenytoin levels. Lancet 1971; 1:62

47. **Bechtle RM, Scherr HH.** Studies on synergists for antimicrobial agents, II. Anti-mycobacterial agents. Antib Chemo 1959; 9:715

48. **Beckett AH,** et al. The absorption, distribution and excretion of pentazocine in man after oral and intravenous administration. J Pharm Pharmacol 1970; 22:123-8

49. **Berkowitz B, Way EL.** Metabolism and excretion of pentazocine in man. Clin Pharmacol Ther 1969; 10:681-9

50. **Berlin A,** et al. Determination of bioavailability of diazepam in various formulations from steady state plasma concentration data. Clin Pharmacol Ther 1972; 13:733-44

51. **Berry K,** et al. Use of Pronestyl in the treatment of ectopic rhythms: Treatment of ninety-eight episodes in seventy-eight patients. Am J Med 1951; 11:431-41

52. **Black Dak ed.** Renal Disease. 2nd ed. Philadelphia: F.A. Davis. 1967. pp. 546-60

53. **Blaschke TF.** Protein binding and kinetics in liver disease. Clin Pharmacokinet 1977; 2:32-44

54. **Bleiweiss H.** Salt supplements with lithium (Letter). Lancet 1970; 1:416

55. **Bleyer WA.** The clinical pharmacology of methotrexate. Cancer 1978; 41(1):36-51

56. **Bluestone R,** et al. Effect of drugs on urate binding to plasma proteins. Brit Med J 1969; 4:590

57. **Bobrow SN,** et al. Anuria and acute tubular necrosis associated with gentamicin and cephalothin. JAMA 1972; 222:1546

58. **Bochner F, Carruthers G, Kampmann J, Steiner J.** Handbook of Clinical Pharmacology. 1st ed. Boston, MA: Little, Brown and Co., 1978. p. 19

59. **Bondi A, Spaulding EH, Smith Dorothy E, Dietz CC.** A routine method for the rapid determination of susceptibility to penicillin and other antibiotics. Amer J Med Sci 1947; 213-21

60. **Borden EC, Rostand SG.** Recovery from massive amitriptyline overdosage (Letter). Lancet 1968; I:1256

61. **Bouchier IAD, Williams HS.** Determination of faecal blood-loss after combined alcohol and sodium-acetylsalicylate intake. Lancet 1969; 1:178

62. **Bowe JC,** et al. Evaluation of folic acid supplements in children taking phenytoin. Dev Med Child Neurol 1971; 13:343 (abstr References and Reviews. JAMA 1971; 217:1272)

63. **Boyes RM,** et al. Pharamcokinetics of lidocaine in man. Clin Pharmacol Ther 1971; 12:105-16

64. **Brekenridge A,** et al. Pharmacokinetics and pharmacodynamics of the enantiomers of warfarin in man. Clin Pharmacol Ther 1974; 15:424-30

65. **Brennan RW,** *et al.* Diphenylhydantoin intoxication attendant to slow inactivation of isoniazid. Neurology 1970; 20:687

66. **Brodie BB.** Physiochemical and biochemical aspects of pharacology. JAMA 1967; 202:600-9

67. **Brodie BB, Reid WW.** In: Fundamentals of Drug Metabolism and Drug Disposition. Baltimore: Williams and Wilkins Co. 1971. pp. 328-39

68. **Broughton A, Strong JE.** Radioimmunoassay of antibiotics and chemotherapeutic agents. Review Clin Chem 1976; 22(6):726-32

69. **Brownlee G, Williams GW.** Potentiation of amphetamine and pethidine by monoamine oxidase inhibitors. Lancet 1963; 1:669

70. **Brunk SF, Delle M.** Morphine metabolism in man. Clin Pharmacol Ther 1974; 16:51-7

71. **Brunk SF,** *et al.* Morphine metabolism in man: Effect of aspirin. Clin Pharmacol Ther 1974; 15:283-90

72. **Buchanan RA,** *et al.* The absorption and excretion of ethosuximide. Int J Clin Pharmacol 1973; 7:213-8

73. **Buchanan RA,** *et al.* The effect of phenobarbital on diphenylhydantoin metabolism in children. Pediatrics 1969; 43:114

74. **Buchanan RA,** *et al.* The metabolism of diphenylhydantoin (Dilantin) following once-daily administration. Neurology 1972; 22:126-30

75. **Buchanan MR, Rosenfield J, Gent M, Lawrence W, Hirsch J.** Increased dipyridamole plasma concentration associated with salicylate administration. Thromb Res 1978; 15(5 and 6):813-20

76. **Burns JO,** *et al.* The physiological disposition and fate of meporidine (Demeral) in man and a method for its estimation in plasma. J Pharmacol Exp Ther 1955; 114:289-98

77. **Busfield D,** *et al.* An effect of phenobarbitone on blood-levels of griseofulvin in man. Lancet 1963; 2:1042

78. **Busuttil AA,** *et al.* Possible cephaloridine nephrotoxicity in a neonate (Letter). Lancet 1973; 1:264

79. **Butler TC, Waddell WJ.** N-Methylated derivatives of barbituric acid, hydantoin and oxazolidinedione used in the treatment of epilepsy. Neurology (Minneap.) Suppl 1958; 8:106-12

80. **Butler TC,** *et al.* Phenobarbital: Studies of elimination, accumulation, tolerance, and dosage schedules. J Pharmacol Exp Ther 1954; 111:425-35

81. **Byers JM.** In: ASCP Seminar on Therapeutic Drug Monitoring - Procainamide. ASCP Spring National Meeting. 1978. p. 6

82. **Casdorph HR.** The efficacy and safety of cholestyramine therapy in hyperlipidemic patients (abst). Ann Int Med 1971; 74:818

83. **Casdorph HF.** Safe uses of cholestyramine (Letter). Ann Int Med 1970; 72:759

84. **Cavalieri R,** *et al.* Metabolic clearance rate of 1-triiodothyronine in man. A comparison of results by single injection and constant infusion methods. J Clin Endocrinol Metab 1971; 33:624-9

85. **Cawein M, Behlen CH, Lappat EJ, Cohn JE.** Hereditary diaphorase deficiency and methemoglobinemia. Arch Intern Med 1964; 113:578-85

86. **Celler M, Christoff N.** Diazepam in the treatment of childhood epilepsy. JAMA 1971; 215:2087-90

87. **Champion GD,** et al. The effect of aspirin on serum indomethacin. Clin Pharmacol Ther 1972; 13:239-44

88. **Chen G,** et al. The anticonvulsant activity of a-phenylsuccinimides. J Pharmacol Exp Ther 1951; 103:54-61

89. **Cheng SH, White A.** Effect of orally administered neomycin on the absorption of penicillin V. N Eng J Med 1962; 267:1296

90. **Chow MSS, Ronfeld RA.** Pharmacokinetic data and drug monitoring. 1. Antibiotics and antiarrhythmics. J Clin Pharmacol 1975; 15:405-18

91. **Christensen LK, Skovsted L.** Inhibition of drug metabolism by chloramphenicol. Lancet 1969; 2:1397-9

92. **Clarke JT,** et al. Comparative pharmacokinetics of amikacin and kanamycin. Clin Pharmacol Ther 1974; 15:610-16

93. **Clarke EGC ed.** Isolation and Identification of Drugs. London: The Pharmaceutical Press. v. 1 and 2. 1975

94. **Clifford JM,** et al. Absorption and clearance of secobarbital, heptabarbital, methaqualone, and ethinamate. Clin Pharmacol Ther 1974; 16:376-89

95. **Clin-Alert.** Anticoagulants—Drug Interactions. No. 103, May 8, 1968

96. **Conney AH.** Drug metabolism and therapeutics. N Eng J Med 1969; 280:653

97. **Conney AH.** Microsomal enzyme induction by drugs. Pharmacol Physicians (Dec.) 1969; 3:1

98. **Conney AH.** Pharmacological implications of microsomal enzyme induction. Pharmacol Rev 1967; 19:317

99. **Conney AH,** et al. Clin Pharmacol Ther 1976; 20:633-42

100. **Consolo S,** et al. Delayed absorption of phenylbutazone caused by desmethylimipramine in humans. Eur J Pharmacol 1970; 10:239

101. **Cooper KE, Linton AH, Sehgal SN.** The effect of inoculum size on inhibition zones in agar media using staphylococci and streptomycin. J Gen Microbiol 1958; 18:670-87

102. **Cressman WA,** et al. Plasma level profile of haloperidol in man following intramuscular administration. Eur J Clin Pharmacol 1974; 7:99-103

103. **Csogor SI, Kerek SF.** Enhancement of thiopentone anaesthesia by sulphaforazole. Brit J Anaesth 1970; 42:988

104. **Csogor SI, Papp J.** Competition between sulphomamides and thiopental for the binding sites of plasma proteins. Arzneim Forsch 1970; 20:1925

105. **Cucinell SA,** et al. Drug interactions in man. I. Lowering effect of phenobarbital on plasma levels of bishydroxycoumarin (Dicumarol) and diphenylhydantoin (Dilantin). Clin Pharmacol Ther 1965; 6:420

106. **Curry SH,** *et al.* Disposition of glutethimide in man. Clin Pharmacol Ther 1971; 12:849-57

107. **Curry SH,** *et al.* Factors affecting chlorpromazine plasma levels in psychiatric patients. Arch Gen Psychiat 1970; 22:209

108. **Davies DS, Thorgeirsson SS.** Individual differences in the plasma half-lives of lipid soluble drugs in man. Acta Pharmacol Toxicol 1970; 29:181-90

109. **Davis JM,** *et al.* Effects of urinary pH on amphetamine metabolism. Ann NY Acad Sci 1971; 179:493-501

110. **de Beer EJ, Sherwood MB.** The paper-disc agar-plate method for the assay of antibiotic substances. J Bacteriol 1945; 50:459-67

111. **DeSilva AJ,** *et al.* Blood level distribution patterns of diazepam and first major metabolite in man. J Pharm Sci 1966; 55:692-702

112. **deSilva JAF,** *et al.* Determination of flurazepan (Dalmane) and its major metabolites in blood by electron capture gas-liquid chromatography. J Chrom 1974; 99:461-83

113. **Dettli L.** Individualization of drug dosage in patients with renal disease. In: Symposium on Individualization of Drug Therapy. The Medical Clinics of North America. Philadelphia: W.B. Saunders Co. v. 58 No. 5. Sept, 1974. pp. 977-85

114. **Dettli L, Spring P, Ryter S.** Multiple dose kinetics and drug dosage in patients with kidney disease. Acta Pharmacol 1971; 29(3):211

115. **Devriendt A,** *et al.* Pharmacokinetics of sulfametopyrazine (kelfizine W) effects of a single oral dose. Eur J Clin Pharmacol 1970; 3:36-42

116. **Dixon RL,** *et al.* Plasma protein binding of methotrexate and its displacement by various drugs. Fed Proc 1965; 24:454

117. **Djerassi I, Abir E, Royer GL Jr, Treat CL.** Long term remissions in childhood acute leukemia: Use of infrequent infusions of methotrexate: Supportive roles of platelet transfusions and citrovorum factor. Clin Pediatr 1966; 5:502-9

118. **Dobbing J.** Faecal blood-loss after sodium acetylsalicylate taken with alcohol (Letter). Lancet 1969; 1:527

119. **Drayer DE.** Pathways of drug metabolism in man. In: Symposium on Individualization of Drug Therapy. The Medical Clinics of North America. Philadelphia: W.B. Saunders Co. v. 58 No. 5. Sept. 1974. pp. 927-44

120. **Dreifurs FE,** *et al.* Serum clonazepam concentrations in children with absence seizures. Neurology 1975; 25:255-8

121. **Dreifus LS,** *et al.* Propranolol and quinidine in the management of ventricular tachycardia. JAMA 1968; 204:736

122. **Duggan DE,** *et al.* The metabolism of indomethacin in man. J Pharmacol Exp Ther 1972; 181:563-75

123. **Eadie MJ.** Plasma level monitoring of anticonvulsants. Clin Pharmacokinetics 1976; 1:52-66

124. **Editorial.** Aspirin and gastrointestinal bleeding. JAMA 1969; 207:2430

125. **Endo Laboratories.** Anticoagulant Therapy—A Selected Bibliography. 1968. p. 49

126. **Espir M,** *et al.* Epilepsy and oral contraception. Brit Med J 1969; 1:294

127. **Fann WE,** *et al.* The effects of antacids on the blood levels of chlorpromazine (abst.). Clin Pharmacol Ther 1973; 14:135

128. **Farfel Z, Iaina A, Levi J, Gafni J.** Proximal renal tubular acidosis: Association with familial normoaldosteronemic hyperpotassium and hypertension. Arch Intern Med 1978b; 138:1837-40

129. **Farfel Z, Iaina A, Rosenthal T, Waks U, Shibolet S, Gafni J.** Familial hyperpotassium and hypertension accompanied by normal plasma aldosterone levels. Arch Intern Med 1978a; 138:1828-32

130. **Federal Register.** Rules and regulations. Antibiotic susceptibility discs. Fed Regist 1972; 37:20525-9

131. **Federal Register.** Rules and regulations. Antibiotic susceptibility discs: Correction. Fed Regist 1973; 38:2576

132. **Feldman S.** Drug Distribution. In: Symposium on Individualization of Drug Therapy. The Medical Clinics of North America. Philadelphia: W.B. Saunders Co. v. 58 No. 5 Sept. 1974. p. 977-85

133. **Fischer E.** Renal excretion of sulphadimidine in normal and uremic subjects. Lancet 1972; 11: 210-12

134. **Fitzgerald JD, O'Donnell SR.** Pharmacology of 4-OH-propranolol. Br J Pharmacol 1971; 43:222-35

135. **Fletcher GF,** *et al.* Cardiotoxic effects of Mellaril: Conduction disturbances and supraventricular arrhythmias. Amer Heart J 1969; 78: 135

136. **Flynn TW,** *et al.* The use of serum gentamycin levels in hospitalized patients. Amer J Hosp Pharm 1978; 35:806-8

137. **Forrest FM,** *et al.* Modification of chlorpromazine metabolism by some other drugs frequently administered to psychiatric patients. Biol Psychiat 1970; 2:53

138. **Gallagher BB,** *et al.* Primidone, absorptive distribution and excretion. In: Antiepileptic Drugs. Woodbury, *et al.* ed. New York: Raven Press. 1972. pp. 357-9

139. **Gallo DG,** *et al.* The interaction between cholestyramine and drugs. Proc Soc Exp Biol Med 1965; 120: 60

140. **Garrettson LK, Dayton PG.** Disappearance of phenobarbital and diphenylhydantoin from serum of children. Clin Pharmacol Ther 1970; 11: 674-9

141. **Garrettson LK,** *et al.* Methylphenidate interaction with both anticonvulsants and ethyl biscoumacetate. JAMA 1969; 207: 2053

142. **Gazzaniga AB, Stewart DR.** Possible quinidine-induced hemorrhage in a patient on warfarin sodium. N Eng J Med 1969; 280: 711

143. **Geigy Pharmaceuticals.** Anturane. Product Information. 1969

144. **George CF,** *et al.* Pharmacokinetics of dextrolaevo- and racemic propranolol in man. Eur J Clin Pharmacol 1972; 4:74-6

145. **Gerhardt RE,** *et al.* Quinidine excretion in aciduria and alkaluria. Ann Int Med 1969; 71:927

146. **Gessner PK, Cabana BE.** A study of the interaction of the hypnotic effects and of the toxic effects of chloral hydrate and ethanol. J Pharmacol Exp Ther 1970; 174: 247

147. **Gibberd FB,** *et al.* Supervision of epileptic patients taking phenytoin. Br Med J 1970; 1:147-9

148. **Gibson IIJM.** Barbiturate delerium. Practioner 1966; 197: 345-7

149. **Glazko AJ, Dill WA.** Other succinimides: Methsuximide and phensuximide. In: Antiepileptic Drugs. Woodbury, DM, Perry JK, Schmidt RP. eds. New York: Raven Press. 1972. pp 455-64

150. **Goldberg WM, Chakrabarti SG.** The relationship of dosage schedule to the blood level of quinidine, using all available quinidine preparations. Can Med Assoc J 1964; 91: 991-6

151. **Goldstein A, Aronow L, Kalman SM.** Principles of Drug Action. 2nd ed. New York: John Wiley and Sons. 1974. pp. 129-355

152. **Goodman LS, Gilman A. eds.** The Pharmacological Basis of Therapeutics. 4th ed. New York: Macmillan. 1970. pp. 314-29

153. **Goodman LS, Gilman A. eds.** Op. cit. pp. 186-92

154. **Goodman LS, Gilman A. eds.** Op. cit., pp. 155-69

155. **Goodman LS, Gilman A. eds.** Op. Cit., pp. 839-73

156. **Goodman LS, Gilman A. eds.** Op. Cit., pp. 1324-8

157. **Goodman LS, Gilman A. eds.** The Pharmacological Basis of Therapeutics. 5th ed. New York: Macmillan Publishing Co. 1975

158. **Gould JC.** The laboratory control of antibiotic therapy. Brit Med Bul 1960; 16:29-34

159. **Goulston K, Cooke AR.** Alcohol, aspirin and gastrointestinal bleeding. Brit Med J 1968; 4:664

160. **Gram LF.** Metabolism of tricyclic antidepressants. Dan Med Bull 1974; 21:218-31

161. **Gram LF, Christianson J.** First pass metabolism of imipramine in man. Clin Pharmacol Ther 1975; 17:555-63

162. **Gram LF,** *et al.* Imipramine metabolism: pH dependent distribution and urinary excretion. Clin Pharmacol Ther 1971; 12:239

163. **Greenblatt DJ, Koch-Weser J.** Clinical pharmacokinetics. N Engl J Med 1975; 293:702-5, 964-70

164. **Greenblatt DJ,** *et al.* Pharmacokinetics in clinical medicine: Oxazepam versus other benzodiazepines. Dis Nerv Syst 1975; 36:6-13

165. **Gross L, Brotman M.** Hypoprothrombinemia and hemorrhage associated with cholestyramine therapy. Ann Int Med 1970; 72:95

166. **Groth U,** *et al.* Estimation of pharmacokinetic parameters of lithium from saliva and urine. Clin Pharmacol Ther 1974; 16:490-8

167. **Grunberg E, Schnitzer RJ.** Antagonism of isoniazid and streptomycin in experimental infection of mice with *M. Tuberculosis* H37Rv. Amer Rev Tuberculosis 1953; 68:277-9

168. **Hager W.D,** *et al.* Digoxin - quidine interaction - pharmacokinetic evaluation. N Engl J Med 1979; 300(22):1238-41

169. **Hambert V, Peterson I.** Clinical, electroencephalographical and neuropharmacological studies in syndromes of progressive myclonus epilepsy. ACTA Neurol Scand 1970; 46:149-86

170. **Hammer W,** *et al.* A comparative study of the metabolism of desmethylimipramine, nortriptyline and oxyphenylbutazone in man. Clin Pharmacol Ther 1969; 10:44-9

171. **Hansen JM,** *et al.* Carbamazepine-induced acceleration of diphenylhydantoin and warfarin metabolism in man. Clin Pharmacol Ther 1971; 12:539-43

172. **Hansen JM,** *et al.* Dicumarol-induced diphenylhydantoin intoxication. Lancet 1966; 2:265

173. **Hansen JM,** *et al.* Effect of diphenylhydantoin on the metabolism of dicoumarol in man. Acta Med Scand 1971; 189:15

174. **Hansen JM,** *et al.* Sulthiame as inhibition of diphenylhydantoin metabolism. Epilepsia 1968; 9:17-22

175. **Hansten PD.** Drug Interactions. 2nd ed. Philadelphia: Lea and Febiger. 1973

176. **Hansten PD.** Drug Interaction. 3rd ed. Philadelphia: Lea and Febiger. 1975

177. **Harth M.** Serum gold levels during chrysotherapy with relation to urinary and fecal excretion. Clin Pharmacol Ther 1974; 15:354-60

178. **Hartshorn EA.** Drug interactions: Antineoplastics. Drug Intelligence 1969; 3:196

179. **Hartshorn EA.** Handbook of Drug Interactions. 3rd ed. Hamilton, IL: Drug Intelligence Publications. 1976

180. **Haynes WF, Elmore JL.** Lithium toxicity. J Med Soc New Jersey 1979; 76 (10): 655-9

181. **Hedberg DL,** *et al.* Tranylcypromine-trifluoperazine combination in the treatment of schizophrenia. Amer J Psychiat 1971; 127:1141

182. **Hillestad L,** *et al.* Diazepam metabolism in normal man. Clin Pharmacol Ther 1974; 16:485-9

183. **Hinsvark ON,** *et al.* The oral bioavailability and pharmacokinetics of soluble and resin-bound forms of amphetamine and phentermine in man. J Pharmacokin Biopharm 1973; 1:319-28

184. **Hollister LE, Levy G.** Kinetics of meprobamate elimination in humans. Chemotherapia 1964; 9:20-4

185. **Houben PFM,** *et al.* Anticonvulsant drugs and folic acid in young mentally retarded epileptic patients. Epilepsia 1971; 12:235

186. **Hoyt RE, Levine MG.** A method for determining sensitivity to penicillin and streptomycin. Science 1947; 106:171

187. **Huffman DH,** *et al.* Pharmacokinetics of methotrexate. Clin Pharmacol Ther 1973; 14:572-9

188. **Hunninghake, DB, Azarnoff DL.** Drug interactions with warfarin. Arch Int Med 1968; 121:349

189. **Ilyas M,** *et al.* Delirium induced by a combination of anti-arrhythmic drugs (Letter). Lancet 1969; 2:1368

190. **Inturrisi CE, Verebely K.** Disposition of methadone in man after a single oral dose. Clin Pharmacol Ther 1972; 13:923-30

191. **Isenberg HD, Shapiro S.** An inexpensive, easily constructed microbiological zone reader - reprint from Antibiotics and Chemotherapy 1958; v. VIII No. 9. p. 466

192. **Jackson GG.** Present status of aminoglycoside antibiotics and their safe, effective use. Clin Therapeut 1977; 1:200-15

180

193.	**Jackson GG.** Proper use of antibiotics. Amer Acad Ophthalmol Otolaryngol 1960; pp. 694-9

194.	**Jefferson JW, Kalin NH.** Serum lithium levels in long term diuretic use. JAMA 1979; 241:1134-6

195.	**Jelliffe RW, Blankenhorn DH.** Effect of phenobarbital on digitoxin metabolism. Clin Res 1966; 14:160

196.	**Jenne JW.** Pharmacokinetics and the dose of isoniazid and p-amino salicylic acid in the treatment of tuberculosis. Antibiot Chemother 1964; 12:407-32

197.	**Jensen ON, Olesen OV.** Subnormal serum folate due to anticonvulsive therapy. Arch Neurol 1970; 22:181

198.	**Jeremy R, Towson J.** Interaction between aspirin and indomethacin in the treatment of rheumatoid arthritis. Med J Aust 1970; 2:127

199.	**Johnson AH, Hamilton CH.** Kanamycin ototoxicity—possible potentiation by other drugs. South Med J 1970; 63:511

200.	**Jori A,** et al. Metabolic effects induced by the interaction of reserpine with desipramine. J Pharm Pharmacol 1968; 20:862

201.	**Kadar D,** et al. Comparative drug elimination capacity in man - Glutethimide, amobarbital, antipyrine and sulfinpyrazone. Clin Pharmacol Ther 1973; 14:552-60

202.	**Kalov W.** Can Anaesth Soc J 1956; 9:22

203.	**Kalow W.** Pharmacogenetics: Hereditary and the Response to Drugs. Philadelphia: WB. Saunders Co. 1962. p. 154

204.	**Kanazawa Y.** Clinical use of the disc sensitivity test. Antimicrob Agents Chemother 1961; pp. 926-42

205.	**Kaplan SA,** et al. Pharmacokinetic profile of diazepam in man following single intravenous and oral and chronic oral administrations. J Pharm Sci 1973; 62: 1789-96

206.	**Kaplan SA,** et al. Pharmacokinetic profile of sulfisoxazole following intravenous, intramuscular, and oral administration to man. J Pharm Sci 1972; 61:773-8

207.	**Karch SB.** Methsuximide overdose: Delayed onset of profound coma. J Am Med Assoc 1973; 223:1463-5

208.	**Karim A,** et al. Pharmacokinetics and metabolism of diphenoxylate in man. Clin Pharmacol Ther 1972; 13:407-19

209.	**Kayden HJ,** et al. The use of procaine amide in cardiac arrhythmias. Circulation 1951; 4:13-22

210.	**Kaye S.** Handbook of Emergency Toxicology. 3rd ed. Springfield, IL: Charles C. Thomas. 1977

211.	**Kessler KM,** et al. Quinidine elimination in patients with congestive heart failure or poor renal function. N Engl J Med 1974; 290; 706-9

212.	**Kiorboe E.** Phenytoin intoxication during treatment with Antabuse (disulfiram). Epilepsia 1966; 7:246

213.	**Kline N, Alexander S, Chamberlain A.** Psychotropic Drugs: Manual for Emergency Management of Overdose. Oradell, NJ: Medical Economics Co. 1974

214.	**Klippel AP, Pitsinger B.** Hypoporthrombinemia secondary to antibiotic therapy and manifested by massive gastrointestinal hemorrhage. Arch Surg 1968; 96:266

215. **Klotz U,** *et al.* The effects of age and liver disease on the disposition and elimination if diazepam in adult man. J Clin Invest 1975; 55:347-59

216. **Klotz U,** *et al.* The effect of cirrhosis on the disposition and elimination of meperidine in man. Clin Pharmacol Ther 1974; 16:667-75

217. **Knouss RF,** *et al.* Variation in quinidine excretion with changing urine pH (abst.). Ann Int Med 1968; 68:1157

218. **Koch-Weser J.** Quinidine-induced hypoprothrombinemic hemorrhage in patients on chronic warfarin therapy. Ann Int Med 1968; 68:511

219. **Koch-Weser J.** Serum drug concentrations as therapeutic guides. N Engl J Med 1972; 287:227-31

220. **Koch-Weser J, Klein SW.** Procainamide dosage schedules, plasma concentrations, and clinical effects. JAMA 1971; 215:1454-60

221. **Koelle GB.** In: The Pharmacological Basis of Therapeutics. New York: Macmillan Company. 1970. p. 460

222. **Kokenge R,** *et al.* Neurological sequelae following Dilantin overdose in a patient and in experimental animals. Neurology 1965; 15:823

223. **Kolmodin-Hedman B.** Decreased plasma half-life of phenylbutazone in workers exposed to chlorinated pesticides. Eur J Clin Pharmacol 1973; 5:195-8

224. **Kostenbauder HB,** *et al.* Control of urine pH and its effect on sulfaethidole excretion in humans. J Pharm Sci 1962; 51:1084-9

225. **Kotler MN,** *et al.* Hypoglycaemia precipitated by propranolol. Lancet 1966; 2:1389

226. **Koup JR,** *et al.* Pharmacokinetics of digoxin in normal subjects after intravenous bolus and infusion doses. J Pharmacokin Biopharm 1975; 3:181-92

227. **Kramer WG,** *et al.* Pharmacokinetics of digoxin: Comparison of a two- and a three-compartment model in man. J Pharmacokin Biopharm 1974; 2:299-312

228. **Kristensen, M.B.** Drug interactions and Clinical Pharmacokinetics, Clinical Pharmacokinetics 1976; 1:351-72

229. **Kunin CM.** A guide to use of antibiotics in patients with renal disease: A table of recommended doses and factors governing serum levels. Ann Intern Med 1976; 67:151-8

230. **Kuntzman RG,** *et al.* The influence of urinary pH on the plasma half-life of pseudoephedrine in man and dog and a sensitive assay for its determination in human plasma. Clin Pharmacol Ther 1971; 12:62-7

231. **Kutt H,** *et al.* Depression of parahydroxylation of diphenylhydantoin by antituberculosis chemotherapy. Neurology 1966; 16:594

232. **Kutt H,** *et al.* Diphenylhydantoin intoxication. A complication of isoniazid therapy. Amer Rev Resp Dis 1970; 101:377

233. **Kutt H,** *et al.* The effect of phenobarbital upon diphenylhydantoin metabolism in man (abst.). Neurology 1965; 15:274

234. **Kutt H,** *et al.* The effect of phenobarbital on plasma diphenylhydantoin level and metabolism in man and in rat liver microsomes. Neurology 1969; 19:611

235. **Kutt H,** *et al.* Inhibition of diphenylhydantoin metabolism in rats and rat liver microsomes by antitubercular drugs. Neurology 1968; 18:706

236. **Kutt H,** *et al.* Some causes of ineffectiveness of Diphenylhydantoin. Arch Neurol 1966; 14:489-92

237. **LaDu BN, Mandel HG, Way EL.** Fundamentals of Drug Metabolism and Drug Disposition. Baltimore: Williams and Wilkins Co. 1971

238. **Lal S,** *et al.* Effect of rifampicin and isoniazid on liver function. Brit Med J 1972; 1:148

239. **Landauer AA,** *et al.* Alcohol and amitriptyline effects on skills related to driving behavior. Science 1969; 163:1457

240. **Lederle Laboratories.** Methotrexate. Product Information. 1969

241. **Lee MR, Morgan DB.** Familial hyperkalaemia responsive to benzothiadiazine diuretic. Lancet (letter). April 19, 1980; 879

242. **Lee WK,** *et al.* Antiarrhythmic efficacy of N-acetyl-procainamide in patients with premature ventricular contractions. Clin Pharmacol Ther 1976; 19:508-14

243. **Leeds AA.** Psychotropic Drug Classification - International Reference Center Network, Psychopharmacology Bulletin, 1978; 14(3):2

244. **Lefkowitz E, Papac RJ, Bertino JP.** Head and neck cancer III. Toxicity of 24 hour infusions of methotrexate (NSC-740) and protection by leucovorin (NSC-3590) in patients with epidermoid carcinomas. Cancer Chemother Rep 1967; 51:305-11

245. **Lembeck, F.** Selected examples of Metabolic Reactions of drugs. In: Pharmacological Facts & Figures, Springer Verlag, Heildelberg, P. 101, 1969

246. **Levi AJ,** *et al.* Phenylbutazone and isoniazid metabolism in patients with liver disease in relation to previous drug therapy. Lancet 1968; 1:1275-9

247. **Levy G.** Clinical pharmacokinetics of aspirin. Pediatrics 65, 2 supplements, Pages 867-72, 1978

248. **Levy G.** Pharmacokinetics of salicylate elimination in man. J Pharm Sci 1965; 54:959-67

248. **Levy G.** Correlation between drug concentration and drug response in man: Pharmacokinetic considerations. Proc 5th Int Congr Pharmacol San Francisco 1973: 3:34-55

249. **Levy G, Yamada H.** Drug biotransformation interactions in man. III. Acetaminophen and salicylamide. J Pharm Sci 1971; 60:215-21

250. **Levy G,** *et al.* Multicompartment pharmacokinetic models and pharmacologic effects. J Pharm Sci 1969; 58:422-4

251. **Levy G,** *et al.* Pharmacokinetic analysis of the effect of barbiturate on the anticoagulant action of warfarin in man. Clin Pharmacol Ther 1970; 11:372-7

252. **Lewis AJ** ed. Modern Drug Encyclopedia and Therapeutic Index-MDS/14. Yorke Medical Books. New York: Dun-Donnelley Publishing. 1977

253. **Liegler DG,** *et al.* The effect of organic acids on renal clearance of methotrexate in man. Clin Pharmacol Ther 1969; 10:849

254. **Lind HE, Swanton E.** 1952 Routine bacteriologic sensitivity determinations in antibiotic treatment. Antibiot Chemother 1952; 11:30-4

255. **Lockett MF, Milner G.** Combining the antidepressant drugs. Brit Med J 1965; 1:921

256. **Lockwood WR, Bower JD.** Tobramycin and gentamicin concentrations in the serum of normal and anephric patients. Antimicrob Agents Chemother 1973; 3:125-9

257. **Loiseau P, Brachet,** et al. Concentration of dipropylacetate in plasma. Epilepsia 1975; 16:609-15

258. **Lous P.** Barbituric acid concentration in serum from patients with severe acute poisonings. Acta Pharmacol Toxicol 1954b; 10:261-80

259. **Lous P.** Plasma levels and urinary excretion of three barbituric acids after oral administration to man. Acta Pharmacol Toxicol 1954a; 10:147-65

260. **Lucas BG.** "Dilantin" overdosage (Letter). Med J Aust 1968; 2:639

261. **Lund L,** et al. Pharmacokinetics of single and multiple doses of phenytoin in man. Eur J Clin Pharmacol 1974; 7:81-6

262. **Lund M,** et al. Serum diphenylhydantoin in ambulant patients with epilepsy. Epilepsia 1964; 5:51-8

263. **Lunde PDM,** et al. Plasma protein binding of diphenylhydantoin in man. Interaction with other drugs and the effect of temperature and plasma dilution. Clin Pharmacol Ther 1970; 11:846

264. **MacDonald MG, Robinson DS.** Clinical observations of possible barbiturate interference with anticoagulation. JAMA 1968; 204:97

265. **Madsen ST, Iversen PF.** Metabolic problems during treatment with long-acting sulfonamides. Proc Third Int Congr Chemother 1964; 1:644-8

266. **Marcus, FI.** Digitalis pharmacokinetics and metabolism. Am J Med 1975; 58:452-9

267. **Martin EW.** Drug Interactions Index - 1978/79. Philadelphia: J.B. Lippincott Co. 1978

268. **Mattila MJ,** et al. Serum levels, urinary excretion, and side-effects of cycloserine in the presence of isoniazid and p-aminosalicylic acid. Scand J Resp Dis 1969; 50:291-300

269. **Matin SB,** et al. Pharmacokinetics of tolbutamide: Prediction by concentration in saliva. Clin Pharmacol Ther 1974; 16:1052-8

270. **Maxwell JD,** et al. Plasma disappearance and cerebral effects of chlorpromazine in cirrhosis. Clin Sci 1972; 43: 143-51

271. **Mazzuio JM, Lasagna L.** Take This...But is your patient really taking what you prescribed? Drug Ther 1972; 2(11):11-5

272. **McArthur J.** Oral contraceptives and epilepsy (Notes and Comments). Brit Med J 1967; 3:162

273. **Mead Johnson Laboratories.** Questran. Product Information. Jan. 1967

274. **Meyers FH, Jawetz E, Goldfien A.** Review of Medical Pharmacology. 5th ed. Los Altos, CA: Lange Medical Publications. 1976

275. **Meyler L.** ed. Side Effects of Drugs. 4th ed. Amsterdam: Exerpta Medica Foundation. 1964. pp. 137-41

276. **Millichap JG.** Anticonvulsant drugs: Clinical and electroencephalographic indications, efficacy, and toxicity. Postgrad Med 1965; 37:22-34

277. **Millichap JG, Millichap PA.** Circadian analysis of phenobarbital induced hyperkinesia in mice. Proc Soc Exp Biol Med 1966; 121:754-7

278. **Millichap JG, Ortiz WR.** Nitrazepam in myoclonic epilepsies. Am J Dis Child 1966; 112:242-8

279. **Milne MD.** Influence of acid-base balance in efficacy and toxicity of drugs. Proc Roy Soc Med 1965; 58:961

280. **Mitenko PA, Ogilvie RI.** Bioavailability and efficacy of a sustained-release theophylline tablet. Clin Pharmacol Ther 1974; 16:720-6

281. **Mitenko PA, Ogilvie RI.** Pharmacokinetics of intravenous theophylline. Clin Pharmacol Ther 1973a; 14:509-13

282. **Mitenko PA, Ogilvie RI.** Rapidly achieved plasma concentration plateaus, with observations on theophylline kinetics. Clin Pharmacol Ther 1972; 13:329-35

283. **Mitenko PA, Ogilvie RI.** Rational intravenous dose of theophylline. N Engl J Med 1973b; 289:600

284. **Morley DC.** A simple method of testing the sensitivity of wound bacteria to penicillin and sulpha-thiazole by the use of impregnated blotting paper discs. J Path Bact 1945; 57:379

285. **Morrell G, Pribor HC.** Toxicology moves toward therapeutic drug monitoring. Lab Management 1977; 15:40-3

286. **Morrell G, Pribor HC.** Therapeutic drug monitoring: Panacea, paradox, or pandora's box? Lab Management 1978; 16(7):15-27

287. **Morrelli HF, Melmon KL.** The clinician's approach to drug interactions. Calif Med 1968; 109:380

288. **Morselli PL,** et al. Interaction between phenobarbital and diphenylhydantoin in animals and in epileptic patients. Ann NY Acad Sci 1971; 179-88

289. **Mould G.** Faecal blood-loss after sodium acetysalicylate taken with alcohol (Letter). Lancet 1969; 1268

290. **Murray FJ.** Outbreak of unexpected reactions among epileptics taking isoniazid. Amer Rev Resp Dis 1962; 86:729

291. **Nagashima R,** et al. Comparative pharmacokinetics of anticoagulants. IV. J Pharm Sci 1968; 57:1888-95

292. **Nayak RK,** et al. Methaqualone pharmacokinetics after single- and multiple-dose administration in man. J Pharmacokin Biopharm 1974; 2:107-21

293. **Nelson E.** Rate of metabolism of tolbutamide in test subjects with liver disease or with impaired renal function. Am J Med Sci 1964; 248:657-9

294. **Nelson E, O'Reilly I.** Kinetics of sulfamethylthiadiazole acetylation and excretion in humans. J Pharm Sci 1961; 50:417-20

295. **Noone P.** Use of antibiotics: Aminoglycosides. Brit Med J 1978; 2:549-52, 613-4

296. **Oates JA, Shand DG.** In: Biological Effects of Drugs in Relation to Their Plasma Concentration. Baltimore: University Park Press. 1973. pp. 97-106

297. **O'Brien JE, Hinsvark ON.** GLC determination of doxepin plasma levels. J Pharm Sei 1976; 1068-9

298. **Olesen OV.** Disulfiram (Antabuse) as inhibitor of phenytoin metabolism. Acta Pharmacol Toxicol 1966; 24: 317

299. **Olesen OV.** The influence of disulfiram and calcium carbimide on the serum diphenylhydantoin. Arch Neurol 1967; 16:642-4

300. **Olesen OV, Jenson ON.** Drug interaction between sulthiame and phenytoin in the treatment of epilepsy. Dan Med Bull 1969; 16:154-8

301. **Opie LH.** "Drugs and the heart: IV: Antiarrhythmic agents". Lancet April 19, 1980a; 861-8

302. **Opie LH.** "Drugs and the heart: V: Digitalis and sympathomimetic stimulants". Lancet April 26, 1980b; 912-8

303. **Opie LH.** "Drugs and the heart: VI: Vasodilating drugs". Lancet May 3, 1980c; 966-72

304. **Opitz A,** *et al.* Akute niereninsuffizienz nach gentamicin-cephalosporin-kombinations therapie. Med Welt 1971; 22:434

305. **O'Reilly RA, Aggeler PM.** Determinants of the response to oral anticoagulant drugs in man. Pharmacol Rev 1970; 22:35-96

306. **O'Reilly RA,** *et al.* Studies on the coumarin anticoagulant drugs: A comparison of the pharmacodynamics of dicumarol and warfarin in man. Thromb Diath Hemorrhag 1964; 11:1-22

307. **O'Reilly SA.** Studies on the optical enantiomorphs of warfarin in man. Clin Pharmacol Ther 1974; 16:348-54

308. **Oyer JH,** *et al.* Suppression of salicylate-induced uricosuria by phenylbutazone. Amer J Med Sci 1966; 251:1

309. **Pagliaro LA, Benet LZ.** Pharmacokinetic data. Jour Pharmaco Biopharmaceut 1975; 3:333-83

310. **Palmer L,** *et al.* Quantitative determination of carbamazepine in plasma by mass fragmentography. Clin Pharmacol Ther 1973; 14:827-32

311. **Parker WJ.** Clinically significant alcohol drug interactions. J Amer Pharm Assoc 1970; NS10:664

312. **Paton WD.** A theory of drug action based on the rate of drug-receptor combination. Proc Roy Soc London SB 1961; 154:212

313. **Patrick WC, Craig GH, Bachman MC.** Diameter of inhibiton zones correlated with tube sensitivities using six antibiotics. Antibio Chemother 1951; 1:133

314. **Pennsylvania Bulletin.** v. 8. No. 8. "Formulary of Generically Equivalent Drug Products." Saturday, February 25, 1978

315. **Peterson V.** *et al.* Effect of prolonged thiazide on renal lithium clearance. Bi Med Journ 1974; 3:143-5

316. **Pfizer Laboratories.** Diabinese. Product Information. 1973

317. **Physicians Desk Reference.** 32nd ed. Oradell, NJ: Medical Economics Co. 1978

318. **Physicians' Desk Reference (PDR).** 34th ed. Oradell, NJ: Medical Economics Company. 1980

319. **Pippenger CE.** AEDL-QC Newsletter September-October, 1977; 1:3

320. **Pippenger CE.** *et al.* eds. Antiepileptic Drugs Quantitative Analysis and Interpretation. New York: Raven Press. 1978

321. **Platman SR, Fieve RR.** Lithium retention and excretion. The effect of sodium and fluid intake. Arch Gen Psychiat 1969; 20:285

322. **Porter AMW.** Body height and imipramine side effects. Brit Med J 1968; 2:406

323. **Poucher RL, Vecchio TJ.** Absence of tolbutamide effect on anticoagulant therapy. JAMA 1966; 197:1069

324. **Raisfeld IH.** Cardiovascular complications of antidepressant therapy. Amer Heart J 1972; 83:129

325. **Ranney RE,** *et al.* Disopyramide phosphate. Pharmacokinetic and pharmacologic relationships of a new antiarrhythmic agent. Arch Int Pharmacodyn Ther 1971; 191:162-88

326. **Rasmussen K,** *et al.* Digitoxin kinetics in patients with impaired renal function. Clin Pharmacol Ther 1972; 13:6-13

327. **Reeves,** *et al.* 1978

328. **Regamey C,** *et al.* Comparative pharmacokinetics of tobramycin and gentamicin. Clin Pharmacol Ther 1973; 14:396-403

329. **Reidenberg MN.** Renal Function and Drug Action. Philadelphia: W.B. Saunders Co. 1971

330. **Reidenberg MM** *et al.* Pentobarbital elimination in patients with poor renal function. Clin Pharmacol Ther 1976; 20:67-71

331. **Rice AJ, McIntosh TJ.** Am J Med Sci 1971; 262:211-5

332. **Riegelman S,** *et al.* Griseofulvin-phenobarbital interaction in man. JAMA 1970; 213:426

333. **Rigas DA, Koler RD.** Decreased erythrocyte survival in hemoglobin H disease as a result of the abnormal properties of hemoglobin H: The benefit of splenetomy. Blood 1961; 18:1-17

334. **Ritschel WA.** Biological half-lives and their clinical applications. In: Perspectives in Clinical Pharmacy. 1st ed. Francke DE, Whitney HAK Jr. eds. Hamilton, IL: Drug Intelligence Publications. 1972. pp. 286-324

335. **Robigon DS.** Pharmacokinetics mechanisms of drug interactions. Post-Grad Med 1975; 57:55-62

336. **Robinson DS, MacDonald MG.** The effect of phenobarbital administration on the control of coagulation achieved during warfarin therapy in man. J Pharmacol Exp Ther 1966; 153:250

337. **Robinson DS, Sylwester D.** Interaction of commonly prescribed drugs and warfarin. Ann Int Med 1970; 72:853

338. **Rosinga WM.** Interaction of drugs and alcohol in relation to traffic safety. In: Drug Induced Diseases. v. III. Meyler L, Peck HM. eds. Amsterdam: Exerpta Medica Foundation. 1968. pp. 295-306

339. **Rothermich NO.** Diphenylhydantoin intoxication (Letter). Lancet 1966; 2:640

340. **Rowland M.** Amphetamine blood and urine levels in man. J Pharm Sci 1969; 58:508-9

341. **Rowland M, Riegelman S.** Pharmacokinetics of acetylsalicylic acid and salicylic acid after intravenous administration in man. J Pharm Sci 1968; 57:1313-9

342. **Rowland M,** et al. Absorption kinetics of aspirin in man following oral administration of an aqueous solution. J Pharm Sci 1972; 61:379-85

343. **Rowland M,** et al. Disposition kinetics of lidocaine in normal subjects. Ann NY Acad Sci 1971; 179:383-98

344. **Royds RB, Knight AH.** Tricyclic antidepressant poisoning. Practitioner 1970; 204:282

345. **Sadee W,** et al. Pharmacokinetics of spironolactone, canrenone and canrenoate-K in humans. J Pharmacol Exp Ther 1973; 185:686-95

346. **Sanders C.** The aminoglycosides: An overview. Syva Monitor May 1980; 1(6)

347. **Scheiner J, Altemeier WA.** Experimental study of factors inhibiting absorption and effective therapeutic levels of declomycin. Surg Gynec Obstet 1962; 114:9

348. **Schering Corporation.** Garamycin. Production Information. 1968

349. **Scherr GH.** A new type of impregnated paper disc for determining microbial sensitivity to antibiotics and other chemotherapeutic agents. Antibio Chemother 1954; 4:1007

350. **Scherr GH, Bechtle RM.** Studies on synergists for antimicrobial agents. In: Antibiotics Annual 1958-1959. New York: Medical Encyclopedia, Inc. 1959. pp. 855-64

351. **Scherr GH, Nelson RP, Gerencser VF.** The potentiation of antibiotics in the treatment of experimental infections. Antibiotics Annual. New York; Antibiotics, Inc. 1960. pp. 321-5

352. **Schoonmaker FW,** et al. Thioridazine (Mellaril)-induced ventricular tachycardia controlled with an artificial pacemaker. Ann Int Med 1966; 65:1076

353. **Schroder H, Campbell DES.** Absorption, metabolism, and excretion of salicylazo-sulfapyridine in man. Clin Pharmacol Ther 1972; 13:539-51

354. **Schuckit U,** et al. Tricyclic antidepressants and monamine oxidase inhibitors. Combination therapy in the treatment of depression. Arch Gen Psychiat 1971; 24:503

355. **Schwartz MA,** et al. Biological half-life of chlordia-zepoxide and its metabolite, demoxipam, in man. J Pharm Sci 1971; 60:1500-03

356. **Serrano EE,** et al. Plasma diphenylhydantoin values after oral and intramuscular administration. Neurology (Minneap.— 1973; 23:311-7

357. **Shand DG.** Individualization of propanolol therapy. Med Clin North Am 1974; 5P:1063-9

358. **Shand DG.** Propanolol. N Engl J Med 1975; 293:286

359. **Shils ME.** Some metabolic aspects of tetracycline. Clin Pharmacol Ther 1962; 3:321

360. **Simon VK,** et al. Pharmacokinetic studies of tobramycin and gentamicin. Antimicrob Agents Chemother 1973; 3:445-50

361. **Simpson TR, Juergens JP.** Biological half-life and rational drug therapy. Hosp Pharm 1973; 8:68

362. **Sjoqvist F.** The pH-dependent excretion of monomethylated tricyclic antidepressants in dogs and man. Clin Pharmacol Ther 1969; 10:826

363. **Sjoqvist F.** Psychotropic drugs (2). Interaction between monoamine oxidase (MAO) inhibitors and other substances. Proc Roy Soc Med 1965; 58:967

364. **Smith RB,** *et al.* Pharmacokinetics of pentobarbital after intravenous and oral administration. J Pharmacokin Biopharm 1973; 1:5-16

365. **Smith SE, Rawlins MD.** Variability in Human Drug Response. London: Butterworth. 1973. pp. 155-64

366. **Solomon HM, Abrams WB.** Interactions between digitoxin and other drugs in man. Amer Heart J 1972; 83:277

367. **Solomon HM, Schrogie JJ.** The effect of phenylramidol on the metabolism of diphenylhydantoin. Clin Pharmcol Ther 1967; 8:554-6

368. **Solomon HM,** *et al.* Interactions between digitoxin and other drugs *in vitro* and *in vivo*. Ann NY Acad Sci 1971; 179:362

369. **Sotaniemi E,** *et al.* Half-life of tolbutamide in patients with chronic respiratory failure. Eur J Clin Pharmacol 1971; 4:29-31

370. **Stern S.** Synergistic action of propranolol with quinidine. Amer Heart J 1966; 72:569

371. **Stoll RG,** *et al.* Determination of bioavailability of digitoxin using the radioimmunoassay procedure. J Pharm Sci 1973; 62:1615-20

372. **Stone CA,** *et al.* Antagonism of certain effects of catecholamine-depleting agents by antidepressant and related drugs. J Pharmacol Exp Ther 1964; 144:196

373. **Storstein L.** Studies on digitalis, II. The influence of impaired renal function on the renal excretion of digitoxin and its cardioactive metabolites. Clin Pharmacol Ther 1974; 16:25-34

374. **Strong JM, Atkinson AJ Jr.** Simultaneous measurement of plasma concentrations of lidocaine and its desethylated metabolite by mass fragmentography. Anal Chem 1972; 44:2287-90

375. **Strong JM,** *et al.* Absolute bioavailability in man of N-acetylprocainamide determined by a novel stable isotope method. Clin Pharmacol Ther 1975; 18:613-22

376. **Strong JM,** *et al.* Identification of glycinexylidide in patients treated with intravenous lidocaine. Clin Pharmacol Ther 1973; 14:67-72

377. **Strong JM,** *et al.* Pharmacokinetics in man of the N-acetylated metabolite of procainamide. J Pharmacokin Biopharm 1975; 3:223-33

378. **Strong JM,** *et al.* Plasma levels of methsuximide and N-desmethylmethsuximide during methsuximide therapy. Neurology (Minneap.) 1974; 24:250-5

379. **Symchowicz S,** *et al.* A comparative study of griseofulvin-^{14}C metabolism in the rat and rabbit. Biochem Pharmacol 1967; 16:2405

380. **Taylor JA.** Pharmacokinetcs and biotransformation of chlorpropamide in man. Clin Pharmacol Ther 1972; 13:710-8

381. **Thomson PD,** *et al.* Lidocaine pharmacokinetics in advanced heart failure, liver disease, and renal failure in humans. Ann Intern Med 1973; 78:499-508

382. **Thorn GW, Adams R, Braunwald E, Isselbacher K, Petersdorf R.** eds. Harrison's Principles of Internal Medicine. 8th ed. New York: McGraw-Hill. 1977

383. **Thornsberry Clyde, Gavan TL, Sherris JC, Balows Albert, Matsen JM, Sabath LD, Schoenknect Fritz, Thrupp LD, Washington JA II.** Laboratory evaluation of a rapid, automated susceptibility testing system; Report of a collaborative study. Antimicrob Agents Chemother Apr. 1975; p. 466-80

384. **Tiitinen H.** Isoniazid and ethionamide serum levels and inactivation in Finnish subjects. Scand J Resp Dis 1969; 50:110-24

385. **Toakley JG.** "Dilantin" overdosage (Letter). Med J Aust 1968; 2:640

386. **Trainer TD.** The effect of the medium on the results of testing sensitivity to antibiotics. Techn Bul Registry Med Technologists 1963; 33(12):209-16

387. **Trolle E.** Diazepam (Valium) in the treatment of epilepsy. ACTA Neurol Scand 1965; 14:535-8

388. **Tschudy DP.** Clinical aspects of drug reactions in hereditary hepatic porphyria. Ann NY Acad Sci 1968; 151:850-60

389. **Udall JA.** Drug interference with warfarin therapy (abst.). Amer J Cardiol 1969; 23:143

390. **van Rossum JM.** Significance of pharmacokinetics for drug design and the planning of dosage regimens. In: Drug Design. v. 1. Ariens EJ. ed. New York: Academic Press. 1971. Chap. 7. pp. 470-521.

391. **Verebely K, Inturrisi CE.** Disposition of propoxyphene and norpropoxyphene in man after a single oral dose. Clin Pharmacol Ther 1974; 15:302-9

392. **Vesell ES, Passananti GT.** Antipyrine pharmacology and metabolism. Drug Metab Disp 1973; 1:402-10

393. **Vesell ES, Passananti GT.** Utility of clinical chemical determiniations of drug concentrations in biological fluids. Clin Chem 1971; 17:851-66

394. **Vesell ES,** et al. Genetic and environmental factors affecting ethanol metabolism in man. Clin Pharmacol Ther 1971; 12:192-201

395. **Vesell ES,** et al. Genetic control of drug levels and of the induction of drug-metabolizing enzymes in man: Individual variability in the extent of allopurinol and nortriptyline inhibition of drug metabolism. Ann NY Acad Sci 1971; 179:752-73

396. **Vesell ES,** et al. Impairment of drug metabolism in man by allopurinol and nortriptyline. N Eng J Med 1970; 283:1484

397. **Vigran IM.** Dangerous potentiation of meperidine hydrochloride by pargyline hydrochloride. JAMA 1964; 187:953-4

398. **Vincent FM.** Fatal Theophylline Induced seizures. Postgrad Med 1978; 63:76-7

399. **Vincent JG, Vincent HW.** Filter paper disc modification of the Oxford cup penicillin determination. Proc Soc Exp Biol Med 1944; 55:162

400. **Viukari NMA, Tammisto P.** DPH as an Anticonvulsant. J Ment Defic Res 1969; 13:235-44

401. **Wagner JG.** Use of computers in pharmacokinetics. Clin Pharmacol Ther 1967; 8:201-18

402. **Wagner JG,** et al. Plasma concentrations of propoxyphene in man. II. Pharmacokinetics. Int J Clin Pharmacol 1972; 5:381-8

403. **Walkenstein SS,** *et al.* The excretion and distribution of meprobamate and its metabolites. J Pharmacol Exp Ther 1958; 123:25408

404. **Wan SH,** *et al.* Bioavailability of aminosalicylic acid and its various salts in humans. II. Absorption from tablets. J Pharm Sci 1974; 63:708-16

405. **Warner-Chilcott Laboratories.** Mandelamine. Product Monograph. 1968

406. **Watt DAL.** Sensitivity to propranolol after digoxin intoxication. Brit Med J 1968; 3:413

407. **Weily HS, Genton E.** Clinical pharmacology of procainamide (abst.) Ann Int Med 1971; 74:823

408. **Weily HS, Genton E.** Pharmacokinetics of procainamide. Arch Intern Med 1972; 130:366-9

409. **Weinberg WA, Harwell JL.** Diazepam in Myoclonic Seizures. Am J Dis Child 1965; 109:123

410. **Weiner IM, Mudge GH.** Renal tubular mechanisms for excretion of organic acids and bases. Amer J Med 1964; 36:748

411. **Welch RM,** *et al.* An experimental model in dogs for studying interactions of drugs with bishydroxycoumarin. Clin Pharmacol Ther 1969; 10:817

412. **Wilkinson GR, Beckett AH.** Absorption, metabolism and excretion of the ephedrines in man. I. The influence of urinary pH and urine volume output. J Pharmacol Exp Ther 1968a; 162:139-47

413. **Wilkinson GR, Becket AH.** Absorption, metabolism, and excretion of the ephedrines in man. II. J Pharm Sci 1968b; 57:1933-8

414. **Wharton RN,** *et al.* A potential clinical use for methylphenadate with tricyclic antidepressants. Amer J Psychiat 1971; 127:1619

415. **Wilson JT, Wilkinson GP.** Chronic and Severe phenobarbitol intoxication in the child treated with primitone and diphenylhydantoin. J. Pediatrics 1970; 83:484-9

416. **Winek CL.** In: Toxicology Annual - 1974. New York: Marcel Dekker. 1975. p. 209

417. **Winston F.** Combined antidepressant therapy. Br J Psychiat 1971; 118:301

418. **Wood PHN.** Faecal blood-loss after sodium acetylsalicylate taken with alcohol (Letter). Lancet 1969; 1:677

419. **Woodbury DM,** *et al.* eds. In: Antiepileptic Drugs. New York: Raven Press. 1972. pp. 170-1

420. **Woods JW, Liddle GW, Stant EG, Michelakis AM, Brill AB.** Effect of an adrenal inhibitor in hypertensive patients with suppressed renin. Arch Intern Med 1969; 123:366-70

421. **"Workshop on Therapeutic Drug Monitoring".** Johns Hopkins University, Sept. 1976, Lecture notes.

422. **Zacharias SJ, Mittler WG, Cooper LH.** The use of mycostatin in media for sensitivity testing. Amer J Med Technol 1962

423. **Zall H,** *et al.* Lithium carbonate: A clinical study. Amer J Psychiat 1968; 125:549

424. **Zeidenberg P,** *et al.* Clinical and metabolic studies with imipramine in man. Amer J Psychiat 1971; 127:1321

425. **Zirkle GA,** *et al.* Effects of chlorpromazine and alcohol on coordination and judgment. JAMA 1959; 171:1496.